From the reviews of *Reverse Your Diabetes* by
Dr David Cavan

'Inspirational [and] amazing … A bible for all diagnosed
type 2 diabetes sufferers!'

11/02/15

'I'd just found out I have T2 diabetes when I came
across this book. It is absolutely invaluable … the
author is extremely positive and so encouraging about
dealing with T2. I thank my lucky stars I came across
this book – it is my bible.'

29/12/15

'If you buy one book this has to be it … [it is] an excellent
book, very clear … if you have struggled with your
diabetes as I have then put the past behind you and start
again!'

26/04/15

' [A] Game changer … my husband read this book and
has changed his lifestyle completely. His blood sugar
levels have returned to normal in two weeks.'

07/12/14

'This book is very informative, easy to read and
understand, but most of all it calmed my sense of fear
after being told I was diabetic. I thoroughly recommend
this book and urge you to buy it, I am so pleased I did!'

10/05/15

'This book in an absolute inspiration from the very first
page … I can't recommend this highly enough.'

18/09/15

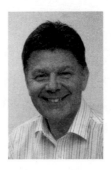

Dr David Cavan MD, FRCP is an experienced diabetes physician who has expertise in all areas of diabetes management, with particular interests in intensive management of type 1 diabetes including insulin pump therapy and in supporting lifestyle change to manage and reverse type 2 diabetes. He actively promotes self-management and has been closely involved in the development of education programmes for people with diabetes, and is the author of 2 successful books on self-management of type 2 diabetes.

For many years, he worked as a Consultant Physician at the Bournemouth Diabetes and Endocrine centre, one of the leading NHS diabetes centres in the UK. He was also a previous Chair of the Education and Psychosocial Care Section of Diabetes UK, in which role he contributed to the development of the National Service Framework for Diabetes.

In 2013, he left the UK to work for three years as the Director of Policy and Programmes at the International Diabetes Federation (IDF) in Brussels. There he was responsible for overseeing a range of projects and programmes that addressed the various needs of people with diabetes at a global level.

In 2014 he published his first book, *Reverse your Diabetes – The step by step plan to take control of type 2 diabetes*, aimed at providing people with type 2 diabetes with the information they need to make lifestyle changes to achieve better control of their diabetes, and possibly to reverse it. This was followed in 2016 with *Reverse your Diabetes Diet*, including 60 quick and easy recipes to help people manage type 2 diabetes. David is currently writing a book to support people with managing type 1 diabetes.

He has now returned to the UK as an independent consultant to work on a variety of diabetes-related projects, while returning to clinical practice at London Medical.

Reverse
Your
Diabetes
Diet

Take control of
type 2 diabetes with
60 quick-and-easy recipes

DR DAVID CAVAN

Vermilion
LONDON

7 9 10 8

Vermilion, an imprint of Ebury Publishing,
20 Vauxhall Bridge Road,
London SW1V 2SA

Vermilion is part of the Penguin Random House group of companies whose
addresses can be found at global.penguinrandomhouse.com

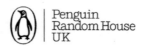

First published by Vermilion in 2016

www.eburypublishing.co.uk

A CIP catalogue record for this book is available from the British Library

ISBN 9780091948245

Designed by seagulls.net

Printed and bound in Great Britain by Clays Ltd, St Ives PLC

Penguin Random House is committed to a sustainable future for our
business, our readers and our planet. This book is made from
Forest Stewardship Council® certified paper.

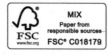

Several of the recipes in this book use fish–choose fish with the blue MSC
label on its packaging. You can trust the seafood with the blue MSC label
has been responsibly caught by a certified sustainable fishery.

Dedicated to
Penny Cavan,
who taught me the value of real food

Get support from Europe's largest diabetes community

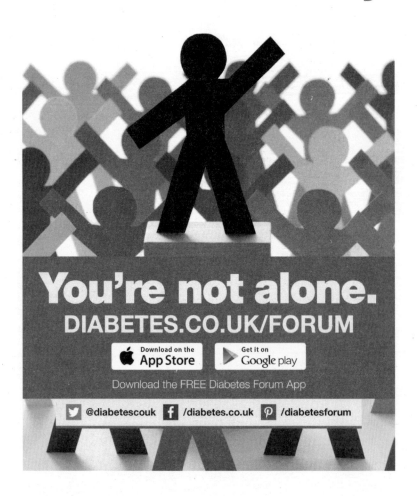

CONTENTS

FOREWORD

*Most people say it is the intellect that makes a great scientist. They are wrong: it is **character**.*

Albert Einstein

What does it take to go against a dogma in medicine when the dogma is wrong? Let us be clear, type 2 diabetes can be reversed. The possibility of reversal is based on much rigorous scientific evidence, yet it is largely overlooked by many organizations in the field of diabetes care. This despite an exploding world-wide epidemic of type 2 diabetes. Not only is the number of people affected growing, but the age at which it affects them is decreasing. Type 2 diabetes in a teenager or even a child was unheard of a few decades ago, but is now becoming common place. When does the care and advice we give to these patients come under scrutiny? When do we admit that we were wrong?

New ideas do not develop because they just sound good. I mean, who would not love the idea of reversing diabetes? The advice needs to be backed by one very important thing: *scientific evidence.* Successful reversal of type 2 diabetes with lifestyle changes has been demonstrated in multiple studies. The uniting factor in all of them? Cutting carbs.

In my work as an obesity medicine physician and lipidologist at Indiana University Health Arnett, I see many patients who have successfully reversed their diabetes. The biggest barrier I see is that most people when diagnosed have no idea that it is possible. Reverse my diabetes? Get off medications instead of taking more?

In *Reverse your Diabetes Diet,* Dr Cavan addresses the barrier head on: **type 2 diabetes can be reversed and here is how**. Helping people understand the why and not just the how is paramount for a true lifestyle change. Much of the advice goes against the standard recommendations, but it is based on science. For this I applaud Dr Cavan. We cannot continue to recommend to people with diabetes that they eat potatoes and cereals and call juice a serving of 'fruit'. Fat has not been the enemy in this disease; it has been the carbohydrates we replaced it with. This book, like its predecessor, *Reverse your Diabetes – The step-by-step plan to take control of type 2 diabetes,* changes the discourse.

Dr Cavan's book does a fantastic job of walking the reader through the physiology of diabetes and provides sound advice on which so-called 'healthy' foods are actually anything but. The recipes provide a solid foundation to get started on a new, healthy lifestyle.

I encourage you not only to read this book but also to buy it for a loved one, friend or coworker who is one of the millions and millions living with this condition. Understanding that you have the power to take control of type 2 diabetes instead of it controlling you is the big first step. Enjoy the book and the new lifestyle which it will help you to begin.

Dr Sarah Hallberg, January 2016

Dr Sarah Hallberg is the medical director and founder of the Indiana University-Arnett Health Medical Weight Loss Program that has helped hundreds of patients reverse and prevent type 2 diabetes through low-carb and high-fat nutrition. Dr Hallberg also holds certification by the American College of Sports Medicine as a Registered Clinical Exercise Physiologist. She has a master's degree in exercise physiology and has worked as a fitness trainer and instructor.

PREFACE

Since the publication of *Reverse Your Diabetes – The step-by-step plan to take control of type 2 diabetes*, further evidence has emerged of the links between certain foods and the development of type 2 diabetes. The harmful effects of sugar on the health of the world's population has been emphasised by the World Health Organization, who in 2015 recommended a substantial reduction in sugar consumption. This was supported by many national and international bodies, including the International Diabetes Federation and Public Health England, who both adopted a policy to recommend that sugar consumption should be reduced to no more than 5 per cent of daily calorie intake. Turning such laudable aims into reality will do much to stem the rising tide of type 2 diabetes diagnoses in the UK and across the globe.

In the meantime, it is important to encourage people who already have type 2 diabetes to adopt a diet that will help them to achieve as near-normal blood glucose levels as possible, by eating foods that will help reduce their blood insulin levels and in turn reverse some of the changes that might lead to their developing type 2 diabetes complications.

Reverse Your Diabetes – The step-by-step plan to take control of type 2 diabetes presented the dietary principles that I advise in my clinical work to help people achieve better control of type 2 diabetes and the rationale for these principles – i.e. the 'what' and the 'why'. This follow-up book begins with an updated summary of the arguments set out in the first book, to serve as a refresher to those who read the book some time ago, and to provide context for readers who have not read it – and who, hopefully, may develop a curiosity to read it in due course.

There then follows a recap on the blood-testing schedules that I recommend, with a focus on testing blood glucose immediately before and two hours after meals. I would encourage the reader to do this exercise each time you try one of the recipes – there is a table to record the results for each one. What I have aimed to write, therefore, is not just another recipe book, but a practical guide to how to use diet to optimise self-management of type 2 diabetes, which includes some new and tasty recipes to enable the reader to put these principles into practice.

Dr David Cavan, November 2015

CHAPTER 1

WHAT IS TYPE 2 DIABETES?

Type 2 diabetes is a condition where the level of glucose in the bloodstream is higher than normal. It usually occurs from middle age onwards, but increasingly it is being seen in younger people. Its onset is usually gradual, without any specific symptoms, and sometimes it is first diagnosed by a screening blood test. However, if left untreated, rising blood glucose levels lead to symptoms such as excessive urination, increased thirst, tiredness, blurred vision and weight loss, as well as infections such as thrush.

The symptoms arise because in diabetes glucose cannot enter the body's cells and so it accumulates in the bloodstream. As glucose is not getting into the body's cells, they are starved of energy and this leads to weight loss and tiredness. As the blood glucose level rises the kidneys try to excrete the excess glucose in the urine. This explains why glucose can be detected in the urine. Its sugary nature provides an ideal environment for the growth of bacteria and fungi, which leads to urinary infections and thrush (candidiasis). In order to excrete glucose the kidneys need to excrete a larger volume of water (otherwise you would be peeing out sugar lumps) and this leads to dehydration, which in turn leads to excessive thirst. High glucose levels in the eyes leads to blurred vision.

Over the longer term, high glucose levels can cause damage to small blood vessels throughout the body, which can lead to the long-term complications of type 2 diabetes. These include damage to the retina in the eye, to the kidneys and nerves, and an increased risk of heart attack and stroke. Good control of blood glucose greatly reduces the risk of these complications. Type 2 diabetes is best controlled by lifestyle changes, principally by modifying diet. However, many people are prescribed drugs to control type 2 diabetes, and until relatively recently it was thought that most people with the condition would eventually need insulin.

THE ROLE OF INSULIN IN KEEPING GLUCOSE LEVELS UNDER CONTROL

In order to understand why glucose levels rise in people with type 2 diabetes, it is important to understand how insulin controls glucose levels when everything is working normally.

Glucose is a type of sugar that is used for energy by nearly all types of cells in the body, so it is essential that all parts of the body have a steady supply of it. This glucose is obtained from the food we eat: all carbohydrates (sugars and starch) that we consume are broken down into glucose, which is then absorbed from the gut into the bloodstream so that it can be carried to all tissues and used as energy. Any spare glucose is taken up into the muscles and liver where it is stored in the form of glycogen. Glycogen in the muscles is then available for later use if the muscles need extra energy (for example, during intensive exercise). Once the glycogen stores are full, any excess glucose is converted to fat and stored in the liver.

Whilst glucose only enters the body when we eat or drink, the body's cells require a constant supply of it in order to function properly. The liver, which releases some of its stored glucose into the bloodstream, provides this service and ensures that just the right amount of glucose is available during periods when we are not eating (for example, overnight). In a person who does not have diabetes the amount of glucose in the bloodstream is maintained at around 4–6mmol per litre.

The level of glucose in the bloodstream is controlled by insulin. Insulin is a hormone that is produced by the pancreas, which is an organ that sits just below the ribcage, behind the stomach. The pancreas has two main functions. One is to produce enzymes that are released directly into the small intestine, which break down food so it can be absorbed into the bloodstream. These enzymes

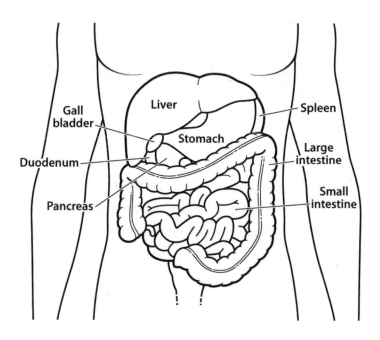

include amylase, which breaks down starch into glucose; lipase, which breaks down fat; and protease, which breaks down proteins.

The other main function of the pancreas is to produce hormones. These are chemicals that are released into the bloodstream and which have effects all around the body. Insulin is one of the hormones produced by the pancreas and, as already mentioned, its job is to regulate the level of glucose in the bloodstream, ensuring that cells get the right amount at all times. It does this in a number of ways:

1. When we eat a meal the carbohydrate it contains is converted into glucose in the gut and passes

through the gut wall into the bloodstream. The body detects that the glucose level in the blood is rising and this leads to the pancreas producing additional insulin.

2. This insulin acts on individual cells to allow glucose to enter them. Insulin molecules attach to a receptor on the cell membrane that opens up to allow glucose in. Insulin is often likened to a 'key' that opens the cell's 'door', allowing glucose to enter it.

3. Insulin also stops the liver and muscles from releasing stored glucose into the blood; this allows spare glucose to be added to the glycogen stores.

4. When we are not eating, the pancreas continually produces a small amount of insulin that controls the release of glucose from the liver. In the liver insulin acts like a tap that turns off the release of glucose from the liver. If glucose levels in the blood drop too low, then less insulin will be produced (opening the tap), allowing more glucose to be released from the liver. On the other hand, if glucose levels rise then more insulin is produced, closing the tap and slowing down the release of glucose from the liver.

The main problem in type 2 diabetes is that insulin doesn't work very well; this reduced effectiveness interferes with both the action of insulin in turning off the tap that releases glucose stored in the liver into the bloodstream, and its role in opening the cell doors to allow glucose to enter the body's cells after a meal.

It seems that the problem starts in the liver, which becomes 'immune' or resistant to the effect of insulin so that even when insulin is present the liver keeps releasing glucose into the bloodstream. This is called 'insulin resistance', and to try to get round this the pancreas produces more and more insulin in an attempt to control the release of glucose from the liver. For a while this may work in keeping the blood glucose level under control, but eventually the liver becomes resistant to even these high levels of insulin and so the level of glucose in the blood rises. Diabetes develops once the blood glucose rises above a certain level – that is, above 7mmol per litre if fasting, or above 11.1mmol/l after a meal.

The progression of type 2 diabetes after diagnosis was perhaps best documented in the United Kingdom Prospective Diabetes Study[1] (UKPDS) that studied the progress of people with diabetes diagnosed in the 1970s. This showed that even with the best treatment available at the time, glucose levels rose progressively over the years following diagnosis. Blood pressure and cholesterol levels were also high, and this study emphasised that type 2 diabetes is not just a glucose disorder but also one in which blood pressure and cholesterol levels can cause problems. This is actually not surprising as high insulin levels have an effect on retaining sodium (salt) in the body that leads to high blood pressure.

Insulin resistance is also associated with high cholesterol levels, and high glucose levels are associated with another type of body fat, called triglycerides. In approaching the management of type 2 diabetes it is therefore important to monitor not just glucose levels but also blood pressure and cholesterol, and where possible use strategies which will reduce rather than increase insulin levels.

THE DIABETES AND OBESITY EPIDEMIC

There is no doubt that in the past ten years we have seen a massive increase in the number of people with type 2 diabetes, and also in those who are overweight or obese. Obesity is diagnosed by calculating an individual's body mass index (BMI). This is the relationship between a person's height and their weight. Normal body weight is defined as a body mass index between 20 and 25. A BMI between 25 and 30 is defined as overweight and above 30 as obese. The precise calculation is to take the weight in kilograms and to divide it by the square of the height in metres. So for a person who weighs 80 kilos (about 12.5 stone) and is 1.83 m tall (about 6 feet), the BMI is calculated as:

- ▶ $80/(1.83 \times 1.83) = 23.9$ (which would be in the normal range).

A person of the same height who weighs 110 kilos (about 17 stone) has a BMI of $110/(1.83 \times 1.83) = 32.9$ (which is in the obese range). A chart to help work out your BMI is in appendix 1.

Until the 1990s, type 2 diabetes was not readily associated with obesity. Certainly there were people who were obese and had type 2 diabetes, but there were also many people with type 2 diabetes who, while a little overweight, were not obese at diagnosis. However, over the past twenty years there has been a steady increase in the number of people diagnosed with type 2 diabetes. There has also been quite a sharp increase in the number of people who are overweight or obese. In the 1990s, it was estimated there were one million people in the UK with diabetes, the majority of whom had type 2 diabetes. By 2014 this had increased to around 3 million – and it is estimated that over 30 per cent of the population were obese.

In 2014, it was reported that rates of type 2 diabetes had reached 29 million in the US, or 9.1 per cent of all adults in the country. That's not to mention the millions estimated to have undiagnosed type 2 diabetes.[2] Rates of obesity, meanwhile, have more than doubled since 1980; in 2009–10 data showed that 35.7 per cent of American adults were obese.[3] And while by no means all cases of type 2 diabetes are caused by obesity, there is certainly a distinct correlation between the two conditions.

This has led to a big shift in the way we think about the disease. In the 1990s people were reassured that they did not get diabetes as a result of their diet or lifestyle. Rather, their diabetes was due to unknown factors and therefore was beyond their control – perhaps it was in their genes. However (and perversely), they were also told that changing their lifestyle would help control it. Twenty years later, with the twin epidemics of type 2 diabetes and obesity visited upon us, and the close correlation between the two, it is abundantly clear that in many cases diabetes has developed in individuals as a result of their being overweight. The message is now very clear: if you eat too much and/or exercise too little, you will become overweight. And if you become overweight there is a greatly increased chance of developing type 2 diabetes. The bad news is that on an individual level this means there is a direct link between a person's lifestyle and later development of type 2 diabetes; the good news is that this readily explains why lifestyle changes can help control diabetes – and raises the possibility that changing lifestyle might help reverse the condition.

However, it is important to emphasise again that not everyone with type 2 diabetes is obese. This is especially the case in many developing countries, where there has also been a big increase in rates of type 2 diabetes, but without the increase in obesity. In many such cases, while body weight overall may not be increased, there is often excess fat in the abdomen (and especially in the liver) and this increases the risk of type 2 diabetes.

THE TWENTY-FIRST-CENTURY PLAGUE

As mentioned above, we are now seeing that this epidemic of type 2 diabetes is occurring not only in the UK and other Western countries, but also in many African and Asian countries, where more and more people live in cities and eat high-calorie diets. This rapid increase in type 2 diabetes has been compared to the mediaeval pandemic known as the Black Death (likely to have been bubonic plague caused by a bacterium called *Yersinia pestis* that is carried by fleas), the spread of which was facilitated by the contemporary living environment of overcrowding and poor sanitation.[4] The plague swept across Europe in the 14th century, peaking between 1348 and 1350, and resulted in tens of millions of deaths. In the case of type 2 diabetes, the cause (or vector) is calorie excess (that is, eating too much), spread by the availability of high-calorie foods and drinks at low cost in the context of a changed environment which encourages an unhealthy, sedentary lifestyle. The rapid rise in obesity and type 2 diabetes cannot be due to changes in our genes, so we have to accept that it is due to changes in diet and lifestyle. The tragedy is that if left unchecked this modern epidemic will prove every bit as catastrophic as the historical one.

Thus if you have type 2 diabetes your eating habits are likely to have played a role in causing it. However, it would not be right to blame yourself entirely for having developed diabetes. It is important to remember that this is a problem affecting millions of people across the world, which has come about as a result of the advances in food production and processing and the overall increase in wealth that have affected, and in many ways benefited, us all. Technology, scientific and social advances mean the world's growing population has access to more high-calorie food to eat. Those same technological advances mean that our physical activity levels are much lower than those of our predecessors. Stop and have a think about your current levels of activity, and those of your childhood, or perhaps of your parents when they were your age. There are obvious differences: such as the greatly increased use of the car rather than walking or cycling; or buying (often processed) food in a weekly visit to the supermarket rather than buying fresh food from a number of different shops, sometimes every day (which often required quite a lot of walking, too). There has also been a significant decline in physically demanding industrial jobs, many of which have been replaced by jobs that involve sitting at a computer all day.

Then there are subtler differences, such as the use of the television remote control that means you have a whole array of entertainment literally at your fingertips. In the old days you had to get up and walk to the television to switch channels; the use of escalators and lifts (in some hotels it is almost impossible to find the stairs); the use of computers, which mean that children no longer need to go outside for entertainment and adventure, and adults can stay at home and do all their shopping, banking and even socialising online.

And at the same time that all this has been happening, food has become ever more plentiful and cheaper. At a time of rising prices and austerity it may be difficult to remember that in the 1970s food was, in real terms, more expensive than it is now. Crisps and fizzy drinks (both high in calories) used to be a treat for children, whereas now they form part of many peoples' everyday lunch. In fact, a packet of crisps is now cheaper in major supermarkets than a single apple. Eating out used to be an expensive occasional event. Fast food hadn't been invented – I remember eating in the very first McDonald's in London in the late 1970s. A friend of mine said they would never last as there were no knives and forks! Whereas previously our high streets were occupied by shops selling fresh food that people used to make home-cooked meals, these shops have been replaced by fast-food chains and coffee shops selling ready-made high-calorie foods and drinks. Even some hospitals have fast food outlets inside them.

Thinking about these changes isn't just a case of nostalgia, but rather it should help you see how our modern environment has changed so dramatically since the hunger that was prevalent up until the Second World War, and how, without much in the way of countering forces, it has inadvertently but inevitably encouraged the spread of obesity. Understanding this brief but important history of cultural shift can help us identify whether we can individually undo some of the changes and adopt a lifestyle more similar to that of our parents' generation.

The changes to diet and activity levels have also led to a big increase in rates of obesity in young children in the UK. By 2010, nearly one in four (23.1 per cent) of all 4–5-year-olds were classified as overweight or obese, and this trend increases steadily through the primary school years to one in 3 (33.4 per cent) by the age of 10–11. As a result we are already seeing cases of type 2 diabetes in children and young adults; this represents a dramatic evolution from a condition that used to be considered as one affecting those over 40 years of age. It also raises the alarming prospect that, for the first time in living memory, the current generation of children may have a poorer health and life-expectancy outlook than their parents.

FAT IN THE LIVER

If we consume more than we need the human body is very efficient at storing the excess energy as fat. We all know that if we put on weight we become a bit chubbier due to increased fat tissue below the skin. This is what causes a double (or triple) chin, for example. We also know that men in particular are prone to carry fat around the middle, the so-called beer belly. This fat is in the abdominal cavity and surrounds organs such as the gut. With the advent of body scanning it has become apparent that many people who are overweight develop what is termed fatty liver, which is just that – excess fat deposited in the liver itself. We have known for some time that people with fatty liver may show evidence that their liver function is affected, not in a dangerous way, but enough to show up on blood tests of so-called liver enzymes, such as alanine aminotransferase (ALT) or aspartate transaminase (AST), whose levels are raised. Occasionally, fatty liver can progress to cirrhosis, which is associated with permanent scarring of, and damage to, the liver.

Research published in 2011 by a team of researchers at Newcastle University[5] suggested that this excess fat in the liver is very significant in the development of diabetes. This work suggested there is a vicious cycle, whereby the excess fat in the liver makes the liver resistant to insulin. This means that insulin can no longer stop glucose leaving the liver and entering the bloodstream (the insulin 'tap' becomes leaky, letting glucose levels rise in the blood). In order to compensate for this the pancreas produces more insulin. However, one of the effects of high insulin levels is that even more fat is then deposited in the liver, which in turn makes the problem even worse. Over time not only does the liver become filled with fat, but so does the pancreas. And just as a liver full of fat cannot work properly, a pancreas which is filled with fat can no longer produce insulin; recent evidence suggests that less than one gram of extra fat in the pancreas is enough to affect insulin production. Although this theory may not explain every case of type 2 diabetes, it does explains how, in many people, obesity leads to diabetes – first by making the liver resistant to insulin, so that blood glucose levels rise, and then by affecting the pancreas so that it cannot produce any more insulin.

It also explains how some people may develop type 2 diabetes without being excessively overweight. As excess fat in the liver appears to be important in leading to the development of type 2 diabetes, and as high insulin levels lead to excess liver fat, then it will be apparent that a diet which leads to high insulin levels may directly predispose to type 2 diabetes. The foods that most cause insulin levels to risse are sugars and refined carbohydrates, and there is increasing evidence from a number of studies that high consumption of sugars and refined carbohydrates is associated with increased risk of type 2 diabetes. Such associations have been reported with excess intake of white rice and potatoes and particularly with sugar-sweetened beverages, including fruit juice.

CAN DIABETES BE REVERSED?

Thus the rapid increase in diabetes that has occurred in different populations around the world would appear to result from generational changes in lifestyle, and in particular from modern diets. This raises an intriguing question: if a person develops diabetes as a result of an 'unhealthy' lifestyle, will they still have diabetes if they adopt a healthier lifestyle?

Until the early years of this century it was assumed that if you develop impaired glucose tolerance (IGT – so-called 'pre-diabetes'), it was almost inevitable that this would progress to diabetes. It was also believed that, once developed, type 2 diabetes was a progressive condition, which over time would likely require tablets and then insulin injections to keep it under control.

Opinions about this began to change with the emergence of evidence from a number of studies in the early 2000s, which demonstrated that diabetes could be prevented. The first study was the Diabetes Prevention Program, in the United States, which was published in 2002 in the

New England Journal of Medicine.[6] In this study people with IGT were randomly split into different treatment groups. The first group, called the lifestyle intervention group, received advice from an individual case manager for 16 weeks on how to change their diet and lifestyle with the aim of losing weight. They were specifically advised to follow a low-fat, low-calorie diet and to exercise for 30 minutes at least five times a week. The second group received the drug metformin and the third group received a dummy placebo pill (control group). All participants were followed up for four years, during which time those in the lifestyle intervention group were reviewed every month to check on their progress. The results were striking: in each year of the study, 5 per cent of the lifestyle intervention group developed diabetes compared to 11 per cent in the placebo group. Those taking metformin were somewhere between the two. The researchers then went back to check up on the participants ten years after the beginning of the study, and although the intervention had stopped after four years, the benefits continued, with a 43 per cent reduction in diabetes in the lifestyle intervention group compared to the control group.

The other main prevention trial was the Finnish Diabetes Prevention Study, published in 2003.[7] This provided similar advice but less intensively (seven sessions in the first year and then every three months for three years), with exercise sessions provided free of charge to participants. Over three years, 9 per cent of subjects developed diabetes compared to 20 per cent in a control group (who did not receive the same advice). In other words, the risk of developing diabetes was reduced by over 50 per cent. The very strong message from these studies is that diabetes can be prevented by losing weight and changes to diet and exercise levels are more effective than medication.

What is often overlooked is that in the DPP a large number of subjects actually reversed from IGT to normal glucose tolerance, something that was previously thought to be impossible. Preliminary data from a number of more recent studies show similar trends, suggesting that not only could diabetes be prevented but impaired glucose tolerance could even be reversed.

The progression from 'normal' through 'impaired glucose tolerance' to 'diabetes' is a continual gradual process, with the definitions of each being arbitrarily set. The interventions described above have shown that it is possible to slow down the progression from IGT to diabetes and to reverse it from IGT to normal. The big question is: can the situation be reversed once a person already has diabetes?

Before looking at recent research in the United Kingdom, I would like to turn to Cuba, a large island in the Caribbean and home to a population of eleven million people. Until the late twentieth century it was also one of the world's largest producers of sugar, with Cubans exhibiting some of the highest sugar consumption in the world. Under Fidel Castro, Cuba became a communist society and a comprehensive public health service was developed that resulted in significant benefits to the island's population; infant mortality rates tumbled and adult life-expectancy increased (both are now better than in the USA). Meanwhile, the more adverse effects of communism led to inefficiencies in industrial production (including the sugar industry) and food shortages. As a result Cuba had to import a number of foodstuffs and many staple foods were rationed. Cuba became heavily dependent on the former Soviet Union for support for its ailing economy.

This support disappeared rapidly after the collapse of the Soviet Union; its disappearance had a catastrophic effect on the Cuban economy, resulting in shortages of both food and oil. By 1993 the food shortages meant 27 per cent of Cubans had lost more than 10 per cent of their body weight and the prevalence of obesity halved from 11.9 per cent to 5.4 per cent.[8] The lack of oil meant buses no longer ran and people had to walk or cycle – in fact, more than a million bicycles were distributed to Cubans between 1991 and 1995. The rationing system protected the population from starvation, although vitamin deficiencies ultimately lead to neuropathy (nerve damage) in over 50,000 people.

This enforced change in diet and lifestyle led to a significant decline in deaths related to type 2 diabetes (by over 50 per cent) between 1995 and 2002. There was also a 35 per cent reduction in deaths due to heart disease. While it cannot be proved that actual cases of diabetes reversed (this would have required a widespread blood-testing programme – not a priority during an economic crisis), the reduction in deaths demonstrates that weight loss and increased exercise had a beneficial effect on the health of very many people. And as we will see later in this chapter, it is highly likely that in many cases diabetes was reversed.

The economic situation in Cuba has since improved and with it greater availability of motorised transport and food. By 2010 nearly all the improvements in health had disappeared, with 19 per cent of Cubans obese and a near doubling in new cases of diabetes. It is of note that the rationing system is still in place, with strict limits on the amount of eggs, meat and milk that is available to most Cubans. However, the allowances for sugar and rice are relatively high, which explains why the Cuban diet derives around 70 per cent of all calories from carbohydrates.

More direct evidence that type 2 diabetes can be reversed has come from the observation that people with diabetes who had bariatric (weight-loss) surgery subsequently regained normal glucose tolerance and no longer had diabetes. In order to be able to measure the effect of such surgery on reversing diabetes it has become necessary to establish a definition for reversal. In 2009 the American Diabetes Association produced a definition of three stages of diabetes remission: partial, complete or prolonged, depending on the duration and extent of the return to normal glucose control without the need for any diabetes medications.

ADA definition of diabetes remission

	Partial	Complete	Prolonged
Fasting glucose (mmol/l)	<7	<5.6	<5.6
HbA1c (mmol/mol)	<48 (6.5%)	<42 (6.0%)	<42 (6.0%)
Duration (years)	1	1	5

There have been numerous reports of the effect of such weight-loss procedures on people with diabetes. In one report 72 per cent of people with diabetes had reversed their diabetes by two years, and half of these were still not diabetic after ten years. There were similar improvements in other aspects of the metabolic syndrome, such as high blood pressure and cholesterol levels.

Research from Italy[9] has described the reversal of diabetes in patients who underwent a type of gastric bypass operation. As is common after gut surgery, the patients were unable to eat and were fed through a drip for the first six days following their operation (a total of 1800 calories per day). What was significant was that by day seven patients had already lost 6kg in weight and their glucose tolerance test was normal. This weight loss and reversal of diabetes could not have been the result of the operation as it mostly occurred before they had started eating, so they were not even using their new gut. It was more likely their diabetes had reversed as they were unable to eat and instead were on a drip, which did not give them enough calories to maintain their pre-operation body weight. The weight loss would have been accompanied by loss of fat from the liver (an important cause of insulin resistance), which in turn would have enabled insulin to work more effectively in reducing the 'leak' of glucose from the liver into the bloodstream, thus reducing their blood glucose levels to reverse their diabetes.

In 2011 a paper was published which described research at Newcastle University that set out to examine the effect of sudden weight loss on both the fat in the liver and on blood glucose levels in eleven people with established type 2 diabetes. They were then asked to follow a strict 600-calorie-per-day (liquid) diet for eight weeks. Within a week, blood glucose levels returned to normal and this was accompanied by a big reduction in the amount of fat in the liver. Over the next few weeks the fat content in the pancreas also reduced. By eight weeks the pancreas was producing insulin normally and the liver was no longer resistant to the effect of insulin – the leaky tap had a new washer. Taken together these changes meant the people in the study no longer had diabetes.[10]

These experiments confirmed the theory that type 2 diabetes is related to the amount of fat in the liver and in the pancreas. What was even more exciting was the discovery that a reduction in calorie intake could reverse the disease process. This is great news because it means that if you have recently been diagnosed with type 2 diabetes then, by reducing your calorie intake and weight, there is a chance that you could become free from diabetes.

The fact that diabetes may return in association with later weight gain emphasises that this is not a permanent 'cure' for diabetes, regardless of lifestyle. Nevertheless, I firmly believe that these experiments should encourage us to pursue reversal of diabetes as the goal of treatment of everyone newly diagnosed with type 2 diabetes. Not everyone may achieve complete reversal, but even partial reversal associated with modest weight loss and lower glucose levels will significantly improve the long-term health outlook for many people.

CHAPTER 2

HOW YOU CAN LOSE WEIGHT

This chapter will introduce the principles behind the dietary advice that I have advocated as means of controlling, and potentially reversing, type 2 diabetes. However, it is important to remember that there are two sides to the energy equation that determines one's weight: the amount of energy (food and drink) taken in, and the amount expended (during physical activity).

So first of all, let's address the activity part of the equation. While official recommendations suggest that we should all be undertaking at least thirty minutes of moderately intense physical exercise every day, this is unrealistic for many people who may not have walked more than a hundred metres at a time for many years. It is also important to be aware that in terms of helping control diabetes, generally increasing physical activity and reducing long periods of inactivity as part of one's everyday life have been shown to be very helpful. Humans are designed to walk, and walking is usually the most accessible form of exercise for everyone (with the exception, of course, of those with a physical disability that makes walking difficult). An obvious target for increased activity is to simply walk more and use the car less. So it may be worth trying one or more of the following suggestions:

1. Consider setting yourself this simple target: only use the car for journeys greater than one mile. That would mean walking to the shop round the corner for a pint of milk. If you work within two miles of your home, think about walking to work. It might be a struggle at first, but as your fitness increases you will find it gets easier (even pleasurable); you will be accomplishing a significant amount of exercise and saving money as a bonus.

2. If your work is further away, consider whether it is possible to use public transport. If there isn't a bus stop right outside your home or work, so much the better, as the walk at either end will do you good. If there is a bus stop right outside your work, get off at the stop before to increase the walking distance. OK, you may need to get to the office promptly, but it's your long-term health we're talking about here.

3. Do you take the children to school by car? Walking with them will not only help your health it will also benefit theirs, too.

4. If you have to use the car to do the weekly shop, increase the distance you have to walk by parking as far away from the shop entrance as you can – where you can usually find lots of free spaces in any case.

5. Sell your car. Forty years ago, it was almost unheard of for families to have more than one car; somehow they managed to survive. If a couple shares a car, only one of them can drive it at any time, which means the other will have to manage without it. As long as it is shared fairly, both will necessarily have to engage in more active travel, by walking, cycling or using public transport.

6. Get a dog. Dogs need walks and they need their owners to take them. A recent survey revealed that 25 per cent of non-pet owners said they never exercised, compared with 12 per cent of dog owners. Taking a dog out for a walk in the evening will not only increase your activity time, it will also reduce your sedentary time.

7. If your job involves long periods of sitting, try to get up for a couple of minutes every hour to break your sedentary time. Are there any tasks you can do while

standing rather than sitting? Is there scope to change your job to one that involves more physical activity?

8. Consider cutting down the amount of time spent watching television. Just two hours a day sitting on the sofa is associated with a 20 per cent increase in the risk of developing type 2 diabetes. Given that type 2 diabetes is reversible, reducing television time should be seen as part of your strategy to reverse your diabetes. You could set yourself a target of having one or two television-free days each week, or only watching television between certain times. The same applies to computer time, especially if you play hours of computer games. If you find it difficult to cut down television time, try to get up and move around between each programme, and try to avoid eating while watching the box, because you will eat more food than you need without being aware of it.

9. Get a hobby. Learn to play a musical instrument – playing the piano consumes calories; playing the saxophone consumes even more. Both involve movement and the use of various muscles. Both will get you away from the television or computer, and should even be enjoyable for you (and those who listen to you, possibly).

10. Join a club. Preferably one that doesn't involve eating or drinking too much. It doesn't have to be a sports

club (although well-managed cycling, running, tennis, sailing clubs, etc., will always supply you with a 'training' routine, discipline and extra motivation when you need it). Try anything that will get you involved in an activity – it's even better if you can walk or cycle there.

In summary, doing anything that will help you to increase your level of physical activity and reduce the time you spend sat down will help reverse your diabetes. So have a think about one change that you can make that will get you walking more and sitting less.

While increased physical activity is undoubtedly beneficial for overall health and can help keep weight under control, the biggest effects in terms of achieving better control of type 2 diabetes come from paying attention to what you eat. There are two main reasons for this. First, for anyone who is overweight (which is the majority but by no means everyone with type 2 diabetes), losing weight is essential to reversing the diabetes disease process, and achieving this means cutting down on food intake, specifically those ingredients that will make it hard to lose weight. Secondly, achieving good control of blood glucose levels is best done by restricting your intake of those foods that cause glucose levels to rise in the first place – that is just common sense.

Let's address this latter part first. In order to reduce your intake of foods that cause glucose levels to rise, it is important to understand which foods are the culprits.

Now nearly everyone I know who has diabetes is aware that foods with sugar in them will do this; however, what many people are surprised to learn is that starchy foods (that is, bread, potatoes, rice, pasta and cereals) also cause blood glucose levels to increase. This is because when they are digested in the body they are all broken down into glucose. People are surprised because they have been told that a healthy diet is one that is based on starchy carbohydrates and to ensure that all meals contain at least some bread, rice, pasta or potatoes. However, some of these foods are broken down into glucose more rapidly than table sugar itself!

Therefore, it makes sense that someone with diabetes avoids meals that are very high in carbohydrates, such as cereal, bread, pasta or rice dishes. This has quite big implications for someone who likes a bowl of cereal every morning (even the 'healthy' ones are predominantly made up of carbohydrate) or a sandwich at lunchtime. However, many people have successfully changed their breakfast to one based on eggs or unsweetened yoghurt, and their lunch to soup or a salad – and noticed that their blood glucose levels have fallen significantly as a result. For main meals, the starchy food should form just a small part of the meal (imagine a classic 'meat and two veg' with a couple of small boiled potatoes, instead of pasta bake, for example).

The experience of many people who have made this simple change is that it helps reduce their blood glucose levels very effectively indeed. And because such changes mean that less glucose is absorbed into the bloodstream, as a consequence the pancreas has to produce less insulin. Insulin is the body's main fat hormone, leading to accumulation of fat in the liver and other organs. So reducing carbohydrate intake is not only good for controlling blood glucose levels, the reduced insulin production means less fat will be stored. This is essential in reversing the accumulation of fat in the liver that leads to the metabolic changes that occur in type 2 diabetes.

If, as well as reducing glucose levels, you also need to lose weight (as is likely to be the case for the majority of, but not all, people with type 2 diabetes), then you also need to find ways of reducing your portion size, not only of carbohydrate-containing foods but also of fat-containing foods. How then can you put this into practice?

- Drink a large glass of water before you eat.
- Use smaller plates and serving spoons.
- Plate up food in the kitchen, not at the table. It has been shown that people eat less if the food is not on the table in front of them, mostly because they are less inclined to get up from the table to go and help themselves from the kitchen.
- Stop eating before you feel completely full – even if there is still some food left on your plate.
- Keep a bowl of fresh fruit (such as apples, pears, peaches) and some nuts to hand for when you get peckish.

When out shopping

▶ Write a shopping list of exactly what you need to buy and stick to it – don't get tempted by special offers or big-value packs.
▶ Do not go shopping when you are hungry.
▶ Avoid buying any high-carbohydrate or high-sugar foods.
▶ Avoid buying processed foods or ready meals.

CHAPTER 3

WHAT SHOULD I EAT?

In this chapter I will discuss each type of food and make some specific recommendations to guide your food choices to best help you control your diabetes. The recommendations are drawn from the evidence about which foods are associated with increased risk for the development of type 2 diabetes. I examined this in some detail in *Reverse Your Diabetes – The step-by-step guide to take control of type 2 diabetes*. Since that book was published, the medical journal *The Lancet* has published a review of the evidence on which foods increase the risk of developing type 2 diabetes and showed that two of the biggest culprits were sugar-sweetened beverages (including fizzy drinks and 'natural' fruit juices) and white rice.[1] In other studies, excessive consumption of potatoes, especially chips or French fries, were shown to be associated with an increased risk of diabetes[2]. What do all of these foods have in common? They all lead to a rapid increase in the level of glucose in the bloodstream, causing the pancreas to secrete more insulin and increasing the likelihood of accumulating fat in the liver.

Eating processed red meat and take-away foods is also associated with increased risk of type 2 diabetes, whereas vegetarian or vegan diets are both associated with reduced risk. A Mediterranean diet (rich in green vegetables and healthy fats such as olive oil, nuts, and oily fish), is also protective. Yoghurt, coffee and moderate alcohol consumption have also been shown to be associated with reduced risk of developing diabetes.

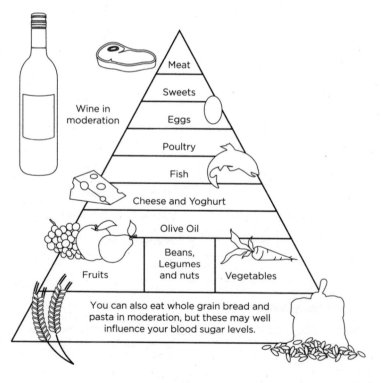

Meat

Sweets

Eggs

Poultry

Fish

Cheese and Yoghurt

Olive Oil

Wine in moderation

Fruits

Beans, Legumes and nuts

Vegetables

You can also eat whole grain bread and pasta in moderation, but these may well influence your blood sugar levels.

So, in an attempt to reverse the changes which have led to type 2 diabetes, it would seem to make sense to cut down on those foods associated with increased risk (sugar, potatoes, white rice and, for that matter, other refined carbohydrates such as white bread or pasta) and to increase intake of leafy green vegetables, nuts and unsweetened yoghurt.

The findings of the *Lancet* paper are summarised in the following table:

Foods which reduce the risk of type 2 diabetes	Foods which increase the risk of type 2 diabetes
NUTRIENTS	
CARBOHYDRATES	
Brown rice	White rice
Whole wheat bread	Potatoes
Oats	French fries
FAT	
Nuts	
Peanut butter	
PROTEIN	
Yoghurt	Red meat
Low-fat dairy products	Processed meat
SPECIFIC FOODS	
Coffee	Fruit juice
Tea	Sugar-sweetened beverages
Moderate alcohol	Excess alcohol

Foods which reduce the risk of type 2 diabetes	Foods which increase the risk of type 2 diabetes
Green leafy vegetables	
Fruit (up to 3 pieces per day)	
DIETS	
Mediterranean diet	Restaurant meals of hamburgers, fried chicken, fried fish and Chinese-style food
Vegan or vegetarian diet	High-energy density diet

Note how some foods, such as potatoes, rice and fruit juice, traditionally recommended as being suitable for people with diabetes, actually make the development of type 2 diabetes more likely. Note also that eating too much red meat (protein and fat) has also been linked with diabetes. It is not clear whether it is the meat per se that increases the risk of type 2 diabetes, or the excess calories associated with eating too much meat, but either way there is an association.

Our ancestors, even in recent history, ate meat once or twice a week at most. Today, in the Western world, many people eat meat every day – and much of it is processed rather than fresh. Buying fresh meat will automatically reduce your intake of the salt and sugar found in processed foods and has the added advantage that you will get what it says on the label.

Let's look at some specific food constituents in more detail.

Protein

Meat is a major source of protein; proteins are vital biochemical components found in all animal life forms, having a role in almost every process in cells. Our metabolism relies on a variety of proteins in a group known as enzymes that catalyse biochemical reactions – such as the action of insulin. Proteins have a role in building and maintaining body structures such as cell shape (cytoskeleton) and muscles. When protein is eaten it is broken down into amino acids, which are then available to our metabolic pathways where they are used to make a wide variety of vital molecules. The human body itself cannot actually make (or more accurately synthesise) amino acids, so we must obtain them from our food.

Protein in a meal leads to a small increase in the production of insulin and a hormone called glucagon. Glucagon, like insulin, is produced by the pancreas and has the opposite effect of insulin in that it raises levels of glucose in the blood. It can convert fat into glucose and this is good in terms of helping burn excess fat; the slight rise in blood glucose is not too much of a problem if your carbohydrate intake is reduced. The body can also use amino acids to form glucose when glucose stores run out. This conversion in itself requires energy, that is, it uses up calories, which in itself may help with weight loss.

Protein is very effective in satisfying the appetite and studies have shown that when people are asked to increase their protein intake they tend to eat fewer calories overall – again contributing to weight loss. As protein is made of amino acids it makes the stomach more acidic. This has the effect of slowing the digestive process so that the stomach is fuller for longer – so you don't feel the need to eat so much.

Meat and fish are good sources of protein, as are dairy products (milk, cheese and yoghurt), legumes (peas and beans) and eggs. For a while, eggs were considered unhealthy both because of scares about infection with salmonella (a nasty bacteria) and because they contain cholesterol. Thankfully they are now deemed to be safe and there are no restrictions on the amount of eggs we can consume. Eggs are a low-calorie food (approximately 150 calories per egg when poached or boiled) and as they are high in protein they tend to satisfy the appetite, too.

For vegetarians it is important to have an adequate intake of protein-rich pulses (such as kidney beans and lentils); nuts and seeds are also good sources of protein.

Fat

The body uses fat for energy stores and to protect most of our internal organs; it is also used to store vitamins such as vitamin D. It is therefore necessary to have some fat in our diet. It is true that fat has more calories per gram than either carbohydrate or protein – one gram of fat has about eight calories, whereas one gram of carbohydrate has only four calories – however, this does not necessarily mean eating fat means eating more calories, as it depends on how much fat-containing food you eat. Most high-fat foods (such as butter, cheese or cream) are eaten in quite small portions and consequently may account for fewer calories in a serving than a standard portion of carbohydrate. Even meat that we tend to think of as fatty, such as pork, also has a lot of protein and its total calorie content may be quite modest. For example, an average portion of rice or pasta may contain 50g carbohydrate and around 250 calories in total. That is more than six rashers of grilled bacon (240 calories) and not much less than a generous 125g serving of roast pork (269 calories).

Fat in itself, therefore, is not fattening just because it is fat. It is only fattening if it is the reason why you are eating too many calories. Fat slows down the movement of food through the gut so that you feel fuller for longer. Thus, like protein, fat tends to satisfy hunger, which can mean you can actually end up eating less overall. Fat also has the advantage that it does not stimulate the production of insulin, which is, as you know by now, the main 'fat-storage' hormone.

Of course, it makes sense not to overindulge in fat, or any other type of food for that matter. However, be careful when buying food that is labelled as 'low-fat', as often it is quite high in sugar instead, to improve the flavour.

Some types of fat are positively good for you. Monounsaturated fat is found in olive oil, sunflower oil (and seeds) and various types of nuts. Nuts have a low carbohydrate content and their fat content (comprising mainly healthy fats) satisfies the appetite – a handful of nuts is therefore a good snack food. The Mediterranean diet is rich in monounsaturated fats and has several health benefits. A major study, published in 2013, demonstrated that following a Mediterranean diet was associated with a 30 per cent reduction in cardiovascular events (e.g. heart attacks or strokes) compared to a low-fat diet.[3] What is also overlooked or understated is that about half of the fat in meat is also monounsaturated.

There is a widespread belief that margarine (made from vegetable oils and several additives) is healthier than butter (made from all-natural ingredients). Standard margarine (as opposed to low-fat spread) has the same amount of fat and calories as butter, and will do nothing to help weight loss. It is true that butter has more saturated fat, which is considered less healthy, but I would prefer to see someone who is successfully losing weight enjoy a small amount of butter as part of a natural diet, rather than someone who remains obese and uses margarine.

Carbohydrates

If you have diabetes it is important that the types of food you eat help reduce glucose levels. The foods that most affect glucose levels are carbohydrates – that is, sugars and starchy foods. So for some time now my advice to people with type 2 diabetes has been to cut down on carbohydrates. To many people this advice is the complete opposite of what they have been taught in the past, and also runs contrary to much of the current 'official' advice still circulating. This is because for many years people with diabetes have been advised to follow the same diet that is considered 'healthy eating' as anyone else, and current advice in the UK and many other countries is to base all meals on carbohydrates.

While this advice might be right for the general population (although I would argue that it isn't), it really does not make sense for someone with diabetes. This is because all starchy carbohydrates and sugars are broken down in the gut into glucose. This glucose is absorbed from the gut into the bloodstream where, in someone with diabetes, it will cause the glucose level to rise. So every slice of bread, every portion of chips, every portion of rice will cause blood glucose levels to rise – before we even consider the effect of sugars in desserts, cakes and biscuits. That is why the traditional dietary advice for people with diabetes so often makes it difficult to achieve its main goal – normal levels of glucose in the blood.

Not only does this type of recommended diet begin to seem quite nonsensical for someone with diabetes, the evidence is piling up that it might actually help cause type 2 diabetes. Note how, in the table above, fruit juice and other sugary drinks, white rice and potatoes have all been linked to an increased risk of type 2 diabetes.

Given the health problems associated with excess sugar, the use of sugar should be kept to an absolute minimum. Indeed, in 2015, the World Health Organization recommended that we should all reduce our sugar intake to around 5 per cent of the total calories that we eat or drink (around 6 teaspoons a day – or about one can of a sugary drink). Ideally you should learn to enjoy unsweetened drinks, but in the real world there are many people who have a sweet tooth and who use sweeteners. The advantage of sweeteners is that they will not affect glucose levels and, as they have no calories, will not directly lead to weight gain or promote diabetes. However, there are fears that they pose their own health risks, and interesting evidence from research on mice suggests that sweetness in food may, in some way, stimulate appetite, regardless of whether the sweetness comes from sugar or a sweetener, thus still leading to weight gain. On balance I think that sweeteners used in moderation are likely to be a better option than sugar, but using neither is better still! So by gradually reducing the amount of sugar or sweetener you use you will retrain your taste buds so that you do not crave sweet foods so often.

Up until now carbohydrates have been divided into sugars and starches, and while sugar intake has always been discouraged, we have been encouraged to eat plenty of starches. As starchy food has to be broken down into sugars before it can be absorbed it had been thought that it had a less marked effect on blood glucose values than eating sugars. However, not all starch is the same. Some starches, such as white rice or mashed potato, are broken down and absorbed as glucose very quickly, in fact almost as quickly as sugar itself. Others, such as brown rice or wholemeal bread, are absorbed much more slowly and have a lesser effect on blood glucose. Glycaemic index (GI) is a term used to describe the amount different carbohydrate-containing foods affect the blood glucose level. Glucose has a GI of 100 and so a food that has a GI of 85 (such as white rice) will have 85 per cent of the effect on the blood glucose level as eating sugar. In contrast, the GI of wholemeal bread is only 53. (Further information on glycaemic index is provided later in the chapter.) So if a high intake of sugars has an effect on increasing the risk of diabetes, it comes as no surprise that a high intake of white rice will have a similar effect.

In order to reverse the processes that have caused type 2 diabetes, it is important to understand what might have contributed to it in the first place. We know that eating too many calories causes people to gain weight and that this increases the risk of diabetes. So part of reversing the process is to lose weight. However, learning that a high consumption of both sugars and some starches increases the risk of diabetes tells us that in order to reverse this process it would be a good idea to limit consumption of these particular carbohydrates.

In *Reverse Your Diabetes – The step-by-step plan to take control of type 2 diabetes*, I discuss in some detail the evidence that reduced carbohydrate intake can help improve control of diabetes. This can be summarised thus:

1. Reducing carbohydrates in the diet helps improve diabetes control and body weight.

2. Reducing carbohydrates in the diet is also associated with less fat in the liver and lower LDL-cholesterol levels.

3. These changes even occur if more fat is taken in the diet instead of carbohydrate.

I have witnessed the same outcome in many individuals since I started recommending carbohydrate restriction a few years ago. The effect of changing the diet in this way is far more dramatic than any medication, including insulin. And some people, who had been on insulin for many years to treat their type 2 diabetes, have even been able to come off it altogether. The conclusion here is that for people who are overweight and have type 2 diabetes, and are therefore insulin resistant, the main culprit in the diet is likely to be eating too many carbohydrates.

So why are carbohydrates so bad? There are two important reasons: first, as we have learnt, the body turns all carbohydrates into sugars that increase blood glucose levels, making diabetes harder to control; second, and perhaps more importantly in the longer term, carbohydrates stimulate the pancreas to secrete insulin, and insulin is the body's main hormone that promotes the storage of fat – under the skin, in the abdomen, in the liver and just about everywhere else. The more insulin that is produced, the more fat is stored. The more fat stored in the liver, the more the body becomes resistant to insulin; the more insulin resistance, the more glucose levels rise, and the more insulin has to be produced – on and on in a vicious circle. Insulin also drives hunger, so when you eat carbohydrates you will produce insulin, which may well make you feel hungry again after a couple of hours. Fat and protein, on the other hand, are much better at satisfying hunger, meaning you can go for longer without eating – so you eat fewer calories and lose weight.

So cutting out some carbohydrates is a good first step to reversing your diabetes. As this will reduce calorie intake, it will in itself lead to some weight loss, as long as the carbohydrates are not replaced with extra fat or protein. Eating less carbohydrate-containing food will also help stabilise blood glucose levels. Note that any change to your diet has to be permanent, so it has to be something that is not so drastic you start craving foods you really like.

Practical steps to reduce carbohydrates in your diet
I would like you to engage in my ten-minute consultation on reducing carbohydrates. It goes something like this:

- What do you generally eat for breakfast?
- For lunch?
- For your evening meal?
- As snacks?

Typical answers will include cereal and toast for breakfast, perhaps with orange juice, a sandwich or baguette for lunch, maybe with a packet of crisps, and an apple or banana for a snack, or maybe digestive biscuits. Followed by a variety of meals in the evening that usually includes potatoes, rice or pasta, which are all carbohydrates, of course.

My first suggestion is to avoid cereals at breakfast and to try a breakfast based on eggs (boiled, poached or scrambled, with or without one slice of toast), or natural yoghurt. I find Greek yoghurt nicer (it has up to 10 per cent fat) mixed with a handful of nuts or seeds and perhaps some oats. And, please, no fruit juice.

Lunch could be a home-made soup (avoiding starchy vegetables such as potatoes and parsnips) or a salad, and while the evening meals can include carbohydrates, the carbs (bread, rice, potato or pasta) should occupy just a small corner of the plate with the rest filled up with green vegetables or salad. Or try a meal made up of just meat and vegetables. So, as a rule, it is best to avoid meals based on carbohydrates such as potato or pasta bake, macaroni cheese, pizza or rice dishes, but you can enjoy them now and again, just accept that your glucose level will rise quite high afterwards.

For snacks, an apple, tangerine, peach, plum or pear are fine (i.e. any small 'round' fruit you can fit in the palm of your hand). Berries are also low in sugar. It is best to avoid eating bananas (unless it's a small one), pineapple or melon on a regular basis. Try to make up your five-a-day from vegetables rather than fruit, but you could also try a handful of nuts, which contain hardly any carbohydrates but contain plenty of healthy fats.

With only this modest information to hand, many people have achieved weight loss and much better control of their diabetes – without additional medication and without more detailed dietary advice. What is interesting is that by following this advice, people often find they are eating more fresh and natural foods and less processed food. This means they are also eating less sugar and salt, as they are to be found in worrying quantities in just about every type of processed food.

Portion size

As a general rule, I would suggest aiming for no more than about 30g of carbohydrate with each meal, although it may be that certain individuals can manage more than this without adversely affecting their blood glucose level. Now this doesn't mean that you have to eat carbohydrate with every meal, in fact it is possible to survive very well (and improve blood glucose control) by having a very low- or no-carbohydrate meal for one or two meals a day. On the other hand, you may occasionally have a larger portion of carbohydrates – as a special treat for example. Note that most of the recipes in this book are up to 30g or less of carbohydrate; much more than this, though, will likely cause a rise in blood glucose levels over the next few hours.

If you take insulin or a sulfonylurea tablet to control your diabetes, it is important that you have roughly the same amount of carbohydrate each day (unless you inject insulin with each meal), as otherwise there is a risk of hypoglycaemia. Learning how to assess and control your carbohydrate intake will help achieve more stable control. Each of the recipes in this book will advise you as to the amount of carbohydrate they contain, and as you discover how each dish affects your glucose level you can work out how much of these specific meals you can safely eat without adverse effect.

Tips to reduce carbohydrate intake

▶ Fill at least half of your plate with leafy green vegetables or salad.

▶ Avoid having cakes, biscuits or ice cream in the house.

▶ Avoid low-fat foods – they often have a high sugar intake.

▶ Avoid sugar-sweetened beverages and fruit juices.

▶ Avoid breakfast cereals – even 'healthy' ones.

▶ Avoid sweetened yoghurt – use plain yoghurt (add some chopped fresh fruit if you like).

▶ Avoid carbohydrate-based meals, e.g. potato or pasta bake, pasta or rice dishes.

▶ When you do eat carbohydrates, use wholegrain bread, rice or pasta instead of white bread, rice or pasta, and reduce the portion size to less than a quarter of the plate.

▶ Enjoy a small amount of dark chocolate instead of milk chocolate.

▶ Use peanut butter instead of jam, marmalade or chocolate spread.

Now you may wish to have some of these foods every now and again. By all means do so, but have them as an occasional treat, for example when eating out, not as part of your everyday diet.

Glycaemic index

We have established that avoiding high-carbohydrate meals will help. This does not mean you should avoid carbohydrate altogether, though. What is important is that wherever possible the carbohydrate eaten should have as little effect on blood glucose levels as possible.

This is where the concept of glycaemic index (GI) comes in. Some foods are absorbed very quickly, which in turn causes the glucose level in the blood to rise sharply. These food types are termed high-GI foods; other types of food that are absorbed more slowly are termed low-GI foods. The glycaemic index of glucose itself is 100. The GI of orange juice is 50, which means that its effect on the blood glucose level is equivalent to half the effect of eating glucose. The table that follows shows the GI for a number of common foods. It can be seen, for example, that a baguette has a very high GI of 95, whereas rye bread has a GI of just 58. Similarly, boiled potatoes have a GI of 50, whereas a baked potato has a GI of 85. Using this information will help you learn how to still enjoy eating bread or potatoes – by choosing types that have a low GI.

The overall effect of a food type on your blood glucose level will not depend merely on its glycaemic index, but also on how much of it you eat. For example, a very small piece of baguette (high GI) will have a much smaller effect on blood glucose and insulin levels than a whole plateful of boiled potatoes (lower GI notwithstanding).

Sweet foods such as cakes, biscuits, pastries, sweets, chocolate, ice cream and desserts all contain sugar and will have an effect on your glucose and insulin levels. Apart from sugar, they also contain fat and anything other than a small portion will have a high calorie content.

These foods do not serve any nutritional purpose and, simply put, we do not need to eat them. In an ideal world they are best avoided completely, and if you do not have a sweet tooth this may well be the best and easiest option. However, they are often very tasty and regularly feature as part of many social events, such as birthday celebrations, a meal out or even that ice cream on a hot sunny day.

Food type	Glycaemic index (GI)
BREAD	
Baguette	95
White bread – wheat	70
Rye bread – wholemeal	58
PASTA/RICE	
Brown rice	55
Basmati rice	58
White rice	64
Pasta – durum wheat	44
Pasta – whole wheat	37
SWEET FOODS	
Digestive biscuit	59
Doughnut	76
Scone	92
Ice cream	61
Mars bar	65

What Should I Eat?

Food type	Glycaemic index (GI)
BEVERAGES	
Orange juice	50
Coca-cola	53
Tomato juice	38
BREAKFAST CEREALS	
All-Bran	42
Cornflakes	81
Muesli	40–66
FRUIT	
Apple	38
Banana	52
Grapes	46
Peach	42
Pear	38
Figs (dried)	61
Sultanas	60
Strawberries	40
LEGUMES	
Baked beans	48
Butter beans	31
Chickpeas	28
Kidney beans	28
Green lentils	30

Food type	Glycaemic index (GI)
VEGETABLES	
Peas	48
Parsnips	97
Baked potato	85
Boiled potato	50
Mashed potato	74
Chips	75
Carrots – raw	16
Carrots – cooked	58
Beetroot	64

Fruit, vegetables, grains and nuts

Fruit and vegetables are generally considered healthy and are often lumped together in health messages. However, it is important to recognise that some fruits contain a lot of sugar in a standard portion and fruit juice and smoothies, both home-made and bought (even if labelled no added sugar), can contain as much or more sugar as a fizzy sugary drink.

For anyone wishing to reverse their diabetes, this message needs to be amended to steer people away from sugary foods. I recommend avoiding fruit juices and smoothies completely and to never drink them to quench your thirst. I would also suggest avoiding dried fruit, except in very small quantities (for example, a few raisins in some yoghurt), because when the water is removed in the drying process it leaves it with a very high sugar content. Tropical fruits such as bananas, pineapples and mangoes are also high in sugar and should not be eaten on a regular basis. Suitable fruits for someone with diabetes are berries (which have a very low sugar content), apples, pears, peaches and small citrus fruits such as tangerines, i.e. whole fruit of a size that you can hold in your hand.

Sugar content of various fruits (per 100g)			
Apple	10g	Kiwi	9g
Apricot	9g	Lemon	2.5g
Avocado	0.7g	Lime	1.7g
Banana	12g	Mango	14g
Blackberry	4.9g	Melon	8g
Blueberry	10g	Orange	9g
Cherry	8g	Peach	8g
Clementine	9g	Pear	10g
Cranberry	4g	Pineapple	10g
Cucumber	1.7g	Plum	10g
Dates	63g	Pomegranate	14g
Gooseberry	6g	Raspberries	4.4g
Grapefruit	7	Strawberries	4.9g
Grapes	16g	Watermelon	6g

Vegetables, on the other hand, contain much less sugar than fruit but differ greatly in the amount of starch (the carbohydrate used by plants to store energy and the most common form of carbohydrate in the human diet) they contain, depending on the type. It is therefore best to consider vegetables in four broad categories: 'fruit' vegetables; leafy vegetables; legumes (peas and beans); and root vegetables.

Salad vegetables such as tomatoes, cucumbers and red and green peppers are in fact the fruits of the plant as they contain the seeds. However, they are generally eaten as vegetables. They all have quite a low sugar content and can be eaten freely.

Leafy vegetables are generally the green leaves that grow above ground on certain plants. Examples include broccoli, cabbage, spinach, lettuce and cauliflower. These are all rich in fibre and vitamin C, with very low sugar or starch content, and can be eaten in unlimited quantities.

Root vegetables are those where we eat the roots of a plant, such as all types of potatoes, carrots, turnips, parsnips and beetroots. These roots store energy for the plant that helps them to survive as they lie dormant over winter. Much of this energy is in the form of starchy carbohydrate and for this reason anyone with diabetes should eat root vegetables in moderation. Some, such as onions, carrots and swedes, are only about 10 per cent carbohydrate, so a usual portion will contain very little carbohydrate. Potato and parsnips are nearer 20 per cent and should only be eaten in small quantities. Beetroot is 10 per cent carbohydrate, of which 7 per cent is sugar.

Legumes are a class of vegetable that produce beans that are either eaten shelled, such as peas or broad beans, or together with their 'pods', such as French beans, runner beans or sugar snap peas. Their carbohydrate content varies considerably and so it is important to know which ones are high and which are low in carbohydrates.

Any that are eaten with their pods are low in carbohydrates and can be eaten freely. Split peas and chickpeas contain about 40 per cent and 50 per cent carbohydrate respectively and are best avoided as they are often eaten in quite large quantities. Lentils and black-eyed beans are better options, but still contain around 20 per cent carbohydrate; red kidney beans are only 7 per cent carbohydrate.

Garden peas are relatively low in carbohydrate, however beware mushy peas that are very dense and can contain much more carbohydrate that you might think. Sweetcorn is, strictly speaking, a grain, but is often viewed as a vegetable similar to peas. However, it contains around 20 per cent carbohydrate and anything more than a small portion will increase your glucose level.

Carbohydrate content of vegetables (per 100g)			
Asparagus	3.9g	Mushroom	0.3g
Aubergine	6g	Pak choi	2.2g
Bean sprouts	2.1g	Parsnip	18g
Beetroot	10g	Peas	14g
Broccoli	7g	Peppers	4.6g
Brussels sprouts	9g	Potatoes	17g
Cabbage	6g	Pumpkin	6g
Carrots	10g	Radishes	3.4g
Cassava	38g	Rocket	2g
Cauliflower	5g	Spinach	3.6g
Celeriac	9g	Spring onions	7g
Celery	3g	Squash	12g
Courgette	3.1g	Swede	9g
Cucumber	3.6g	Sweetcorn	19g
Kale	9g	Sweet potato	20g
Leek	14g	Turnip	6g
Lettuce	2.9g	Watercress	1.3g

Grains are foods that come from wheat, rice, oats, barley or other cereals. They are rich in carbohydrates and can be found in all types of bread, pasta, rice and breakfast cereals. Grains are classified either as whole grains or refined grains. Whole grains are recommended because they contain dietary fibre, iron and a number of B vitamins. Examples include wholemeal flour, brown rice or wholemeal pasta. Refined grains have been milled, a process that removes the fibre, iron and vitamins, to produce white flour, white rice or pasta. When the fibre is removed by way of the refining process it increases the glycaemic index, meaning these products will have a greater effect on blood glucose levels. For people with diabetes, wholegrains are to be preferred. However, some people with irritable bowel syndrome may not be able to eat wholegrains that contain insoluble fibre. It is also important to remember that a large portion of rice or pasta will have a big effect on your glucose and insulin levels, regardless of the type; the wholemeal variety will simply lead to a more prolonged effect. The advice, therefore, is to eat and enjoy the types of bread, rice or pasta that you like, but to keep to small portions, especially if it is made with refined ingredients (e.g. white bread or rice).

Nuts and seeds

Nuts and seeds contain protein and healthy plant fats with relatively little carbohydrate. They are quite high in energy and so a small portion, such as a handful of nuts, is a good option for a snack and will satisfy hunger, but will have no significant effect on your blood glucose or insulin levels. Nuts or seeds can also be added to natural yoghurt to make a nutritious, unprocessed alternative to breakfast cereal. Beware, though, that even a moderate portion will contain many calories – a small 50g pack of unsalted raw peanuts, for example, contains nearly 300 calories.

To summarise: in order to help reverse your diabetes it is important not to lump all fruit and vegetables together into one category, as current recommendations do. Focus on eating those that will have the least effect on your glucose or insulin levels, such as:

▶ Berries
▶ Leafy and salad vegetables
▶ Mangetout and French or runner beans.

The following can be eaten in moderation:

▶ Apples, pears, citrus fruit, peaches
▶ Carrots and swedes
▶ Peas, lentils and kidney beans
▶ Seeds and nuts.

These should be eaten in small quantities only:

▶ Banana, pineapple, melon
▶ Potatoes, parsnips and chickpeas
▶ Bread, rice, pasta and breakfast cereals.

Drinks

Drinks are an important part of life and many are very enjoyable. However, strictly speaking, we only need one and that is water. (Or perhaps two, if you include breast milk for babies.) It is recommended that we drink at least 1.2 litres a day, which is six average-sized glasses or cups.

It doesn't have to be plain water and can include other drinks such as unsweetened tea and 'normal' coffee (i.e. not a high-calorie large cappuccino).

Water is undoubtedly the best drink for quenching thirst – it is cheap, natural and contains no calories. Drinking a glass of water before you eat is said by some to help you lose weight because it makes your stomach fuller so you feel you don't need to eat so much.

Fruit juice and smoothies, whether home-made or processed, should be avoided altogether. However, if you really enjoy these have a small glass and enjoy the texture and flavour. Don't drink them to quench your thirst or to satisfy hunger.

Tea and coffee are an important part of daily life. Drinking a few cups of tea or coffee is unlikely to pose a problem – in fact, a few cups of coffee a day may actually be beneficial for your diabetes, although excessive coffee consumption may impair the effect of insulin (i.e. cause worse insulin resistance). Other hot drinks, such as drinking chocolate or malted drinks, contain a significant amount of sugar and should generally be avoided.

People with diabetes can drink alcoholic drinks but need to consider the effect they have on blood glucose levels. Alcohol itself can lower blood glucose, and for people treated with insulin in particular, consumption of a large amount of alcohol can lead to glucose levels falling too low. For people with type 2 diabetes, the main concern is the effect of specific drinks in increasing glucose levels and the calories from both sugar and alcohol in causing weight gain and fat accumulation.

Beer contains carbohydrates in the form of starch and a very small amount of sugar (in the form of maltose). The amount varies according to the type, but on average a pint of beer may contain about 10g of carbohydrates. Anything more than one pint will therefore have a definite effect on raising blood glucose levels. Cider is generally sweeter, up to 20g of sugar per pint, and is best avoided altogether. Most wine is generally low in carbohydrates, with the exception of sweet white wine. Some liqueurs are very sweet: Baileys is about 20 per cent sugar and Amaretto 60 per cent! Anything other than a very small shot will definitely increase your glucose level. Spirits, on the other hand, are generally free from carbohydrates and will have no effect on raising your glucose level, but they are often drunk with a sugar-containing mixer. Also beware that low-alcohol beers and wines generally have a high carbohydrate content.

If you do want to drink alcohol, I would recommend low-carbohydrate drinks such as dry white wine, red wine or spirits (without sweet mixers) in order to minimise the effect on blood glucose levels. Stopping drinking alcohol altogether will help with weight loss, due to the calories it contains, and you may wish to consider this for a period if you would like to lose a large amount of weight.

What Should I Eat?

Type of drink with standard serving size (% alcohol by volume)	Grams of carbohydrate	Units of alcohol
Vodka 25ml single measure (40%)	0	1
Gin, Bacardi 50ml double (40%) with slimline mixer	0	2
Cognac 50ml double measure (40%)	0	2
Pilsner beer 330ml bottle (5%)	0	2
White wine 175ml regular glass (12.5%)	5	2
Red wine 250ml large glass (15%)	5	4
Port, sherry, vermouth 50ml glass (15–20%)	5	1
Beer 1 pint (3–4%)	10	2
Lager 330ml bottle (5%)	10	2
Liqueur (Baileys Irish cream, Tia Maria) 50ml	15	1
Stout (Guinness) 1 pint (4%)	15	2
Cider 1 pint (5%)	20	2½
Bacardi Breezer, Smirnoff Ice 275ml bottle (5%)	25–30	1½
Double vodka Red Bull	25	2
Vintage cider 500ml bottle (8%)	40	4
Low-alcohol beer 330ml bottle (less than 1%)	20	trace
Low-alcohol wine 175ml glass (less than 1%)	20	trace
Cola, lemonade, fruit juice 150ml as mixer	15	0
Red Bull 200ml can	25	0
J20 330ml bottle	35	0
Mineral water, soda water, slimline or diet drinks	0	0

CHAPTER 4

MONITORING YOUR BLOOD GLUCOSE LEVELS

The aim of managing type 2 diabetes is to achieve blood glucose values that are as near normal as possible. If you are trying to adapt your lifestyle to achieve better control of your diabetes, it is important to know whether the changes you make are having the desired effect. While an HbA1c test is useful in showing the overall level of glucose control over the previous six to eight weeks, the only way of knowing how your lifestyle, and especially the meals you eat, affects your glucose levels is to do blood tests. There are several types of test strip available for this purpose, as well as meters that display the result within a few seconds. In this chapter I will summarise how you can use blood testing to monitor type 2 diabetes.

The disadvantage of blood testing is that you need to prick your finger to get some blood out. This means using a device to make a small pinprick, which some people may find quite uncomfortable at first. It can also be quite inconvenient, especially for people who work in dirty environments, for example, or who handle food, or who are not readily able to wash their hands (which is a requirement for an accurate result). Despite these drawbacks, blood testing provides an accurate record of the blood glucose level at the precise time that the test was done. This means it can be very useful not only in checking the fasting glucose level, but also in seeing what effect eating a meal has on the glucose level. For anyone who wishes to monitor their diabetes control on a regular basis, blood testing is the only option.

However, over the past ten years there has been a lot of controversy about the usefulness of blood testing in people with type 2 diabetes. It is recognised that it is essential for anyone who is on insulin, but apart from that it is often not recommended. Indeed, in some areas of the country GPs will not prescribe blood test strips to people with type 2 diabetes. This bias against blood testing has been fuelled by the fact that test strips are relatively expensive (about 30p each), and they do not often seem to help improve diabetes control. In fact, there was a study performed in Northern Ireland a few years ago that suggested that doing regular blood tests was associated with increased depression in people with type 2 diabetes who were being treated with diet or tablets.

More recent studies suggest that using blood tests can have positive effects on both diabetes control and on well-being. The key here is not just blood testing but structured testing. In my book, *Reverse Your Diabetes – The step-by-step plan to take control of type 2 diabetes*, I explained three ways in which structured blood testing can be used. These are summarised below:

▶ The first is to check the level of blood glucose on a fasting day once a week (for example every Wednesday). This is what I would call maintenance testing for people whose diabetes is already well controlled. It can also be used alongside the second type of testing described below. As long as the test is within the desired range (usually 4–6mmol/l) and the HbA1c is within range, or coming down towards the target, then no further tests need be done. If on a particular week the fasting level is raised, then the test can be repeated for the next two days; if all three tests are high, more intensive testing may be necessary, as described below.

▶ The second type of structured testing is paired mealtime testing, where a person checks their blood glucose just before a meal and two hours afterwards. Ideally the glucose level should stay about the same, or rise by at most 2–3mmol/l. Performing a paired test for one meal, once or twice a week, has been shown to help people achieve better control of their diabetes. Using such results, a person can assess how a particular meal, such as one of the recipes in this book, affects his or her blood glucose level. If a recipe leads to a big rise in blood glucose after two hours, then next time you make it you know that you should reduce the amount of carbohydrate in it. Once a person has identified that they can eat a particular meal, or portion of carbohydrate (such as rice), without adversely affecting their glucose control, they no longer need to test whenever they eat that same meal or portion.

As you try the recipes in this book, I would suggest performing a paired test, to assess their effect. For each recipe there is space for you to record your blood glucose before and two hours after the meal, and to make any notes about whether and how you changed the recipe the next time you used it, as in the example below:

Date	Time	Blood glucose level before meal	Blood glucose level 2 hours after meal	After-meal blood glucose on target (y/n)?	Notes, e.g. any changes made to recipe or portion size
2/3	1230	6.8	11.2	N	no second helping

Note, the blood glucose level after the meal should be no more than 2–3mmol/l higher than it was before the meal.

▶ The third type of structured testing is a seven-point profile. This means doing a blood test before and after the three main meals of the day and also at bedtime. This can be done to see if any further dietary changes need to be made if a person's weekly fasting tests are getting higher. It has also been shown that performing a seven-point profile for three consecutive days once every three months can help people with type 2 diabetes, who are treated with diet or tablets, to achieve better overall control of their diabetes. Indeed, it would appear that just doing the tests has an effect on a person's behaviour, and often the results for the third day are lower than those of the first. This is probably because seeing any high values on the first day leads the person, consciously or not, to make changes to their diet. This particular type of testing has not only been shown to help people achieve better control of their diabetes, but also to increase their well-being. This is in contrast to studies of unstructured testing, and is likely to be a result of the fact that a structured approach enables the person to make changes, which lead to better glucose control.

If you are doing a three-day profile I would recommend you use a form such as the one below (also found at the end of the book), in order to record your readings. If you are using recipes from the book during the three days that you are doing the profile, you could also record the page number so that you can readily review the effects of those specific meals on your glucose levels.

Reverse Your Diabetes Diet

	Meal/recipe page	Pre-meal blood glucose	Post-meal blood glucose	Notes
Day 1	Date:			
Breakfast				
Lunch				
Dinner				
Bedtime				
Day 2	Date:			
Breakfast				
Lunch				
Dinner				
Bedtime				
Day 3	Date:			
Breakfast				
Lunch				
Dinner				
Bedtime				

If you are newly diagnosed with type 2 diabetes, I would recommend the once-a-week maintenance test for the first four weeks or so, as this is sufficient to show glucose levels falling as dietary changes are made. Once the fasting level is below 10mmol/l, paired testing can be introduced – for example, for two different meals a week – to enable you to learn the effect of different meals on your glucose control. A three-day, seven-point profile could then be performed after three months, in order to help you and your doctor assess your overall progress. Once glucose levels are approaching the normal range, a long-term testing strategy might include a fasting test every two weeks, occasional paired mealtime tests (say once a week) and a three-day profile every three months. Using this strategy, a pot of 50 test strips would last about three months.

SIMPLE BREAKFASTS
AND BRUNCHES

SCRAMBLED EGGS

Serves 1
2 eggs
½ tbsp unsalted butter
a good pinch of sea salt
½ tbsp crème fraîche
freshly ground black pepper, to taste (optional)

Start by breaking the eggs into a small, heavy-based saucepan and then add the butter and salt.

Put the pan on a medium heat and stir the eggs and butter together with a small wooden spoon.

Now leave the saucepan for a good 10 seconds before giving everything another stir. As the eggs start to set, remove and return them to the heat while stirring continuously until they're nearly cooked to your preferred consistency.

Take the pan off the heat just before the eggs are done and stir in the crème fraîche and a grind of black pepper, if you like. Serve immediately.

Nutrition Facts (per serving)
Calories 208 | Total Fat 8.5g | Sat Fat 7.2g | Carbs 1g | Fibre 0g | Protein 13g

Date	Time	Blood glucose level before meal	Blood glucose level 2 hours after meal	After-meal blood glucose on target (y/n)?	Notes, e.g. any changes made to recipe or portion size

SMOKED SALMON WITH CHIVE SCRAMBLED EGGS

Serves 4

200g (7oz) smoked salmon

4 x Scrambled Eggs (see page 69)

small bunch of chives, finely chopped

2 tbsp crème fraîche, to serve

Remove the smoked salmon from the fridge and allow it come to room temperature for about 30 minutes.

Scramble your eggs following the recipe on page 69, folding in most of the chopped chives just as the eggs begin to set.

Place the salmon on four serving plates, each along with a helping of eggs. Dollop ½ tablespoon of crème fraîche on the top of each portion of salmon and scatter the remaining chives over everything.

Tips

You can, of course, use other green herbs in place of the chives – give tarragon, oregano or parsley a try.

For a Scandinavian twist, use gravlax (a Norwegian version of salmon cured in sugar, salt and dill) in place of the smoked salmon and serve with a small piece of rye bread.

Nutrition Facts (per serving)

Calories 293 | Total Fat 12g | Sat Fat 7.5g | Carbs 1g | Fibre 0g | Protein 22g

Reverse Your Diabetes Diet

Date	Time	Blood glucose level before meal	Blood glucose level 2 hours after meal	After-meal blood glucose on target (y/n)?	Notes, e.g. any changes made to recipe or portion size

GIANCARLO CALDESI'S FRIED EGGS WITH TOMATO SAUCE

Owner of London's Caffé Caldesi, Giancarlo Caldesi has a passion for Italian cooking and has been a highly regarded restaurateur since 1986. Three years ago, Giancarlo was diagnosed with type 2 diabetes. Unsure what the diagnosis meant, he researched the condition and soon understood that lifestyle and dietary changes would be important in managing the disease. Today, after adopting a low-carb diet and cutting out all added sugar, Giancarlo no longer has diabetes.

This is a recipe that has been handed down across the Caldesi generations and was something that Giancarlo's father regularly cooked for him as a boy.

A word about sourdough bread: it has become an increasingly fashionable loaf in the kitchen, which is hardly surprising given its superior taste which arises out of the lactic and acetic acids that ferment the dough. It also has significant health benefits, including the same acids that slow down the rate at which glucose is released into the bloodstream and lowers the bread's glycaemic index.

Serves 4

1 tbsp ground black pepper, plus extra to serve
2 garlic cloves, lightly crushed with the back of a knife,
*   peeled and torn into a few pieces*
100ml (3½fl oz) extra-virgin olive oil

½ medium onion, finely chopped (about 160g/5½oz)
2 x 400g (14oz) cans chopped tomatoes
8g (¼oz) salt, plus extra to serve
8 large eggs
4 slices of sourdough bread

Grind the pepper into a deep heavy-based pan, add the garlic and all of the oil and cook on a very gentle heat for about 1 minute until you can detect the lovely garlic and pepper aromas flavouring the oil. Do not let the garlic brown. Add the onion to the pan and stir to coat in the oil. Cover the pan with a lid and sweat the onion for 5 minutes on a gentle heat until it becomes translucent but has not browned. Now add the tomatoes with all of their juices and the salt. Give everything a good stir and bring to a very gentle simmer. Cook with the lid off for about 40 minutes.

When the tomato sauce is ready, transfer a quarter of it to a medium-sized frying pan and carefully crack two eggs into the centre. Sprinkle the whites with a small pinch of salt and a grind of pepper. Cook on a medium heat with the lid on for about 5 minutes or until the eggs are cooked to your preferred consistency. Repeat for each of the remaining three servings, or use more than one frying pan.

While the eggs are cooking, toast 4 slices of sourdough bread and place on 4 warmed serving plates Transfer the contents of the pan to the plates, covering the toast. Serve immediately.

Nutrition Facts (per serving)

Calories 396 | Total Fat 34g | Sat Fat 13g | Carbs 10g | Fibre 4g | Protein 15g

Date	Time	Blood glucose level before meal	Blood glucose level 2 hours after meal	After-meal blood glucose on target (y/n)?	Notes, e.g. any changes made to recipe or portion size

POACHED EGGS WITH VEGETABLES

Achieving perfect-every-time poached eggs takes a bit of practice. Some suggest the eggs should be cracked into a ramekin before tipping into the simmering water, but if you have the dexterity, cracking an egg straight into the swirling water and watching the albumen (egg white) form a translucent 'shell' around the yolk is a strangely satisfying experience.

Serves 4

4 tbsp extra-virgin olive oil

1 aubergine, trimmed and cut into ½cm (¼in) slices

1 small red onion, quartered

2 courgettes, trimmed and cut into ½cm (¼inch) slices

4 medium tomatoes, skinned, deseeded and chopped
(or a can of plum tomatoes, drained)

2 tbsp white wine vinegar

4 eggs

salt, to taste

Heat 3 tablespoons of the oil in a heavy-based pan, add the aubergine and cook on both sides until they have taken on a lovely golden brown colour. Remove from the pan and set aside.

Add the remainder of the oil to the same pan and cook the onion quarters until they are brown on all sides (a pair of kitchen tongs will help enormously), then return the aubergine to the pan along with the courgettes and tomatoes. Cook for about 30 minutes with the lid on, stirring from time to time.

As the vegetable cooking time nears the end, poach your eggs. Bring a pan of salted water to the boil then lower the heat to a steady simmering. Add the white wine vinegar and swirl the water with a fork. Break each egg into the pan and watch as the white of the egg wraps itself around the yolk (hopefully). Poach the eggs for 3–4 minutes. Remove with a slotted spoon ensuring you drain each egg well. Serve with a helping of the hot vegetables.

Nutrition Facts (per serving)
Calories 280 | Total Fat 15g | Sat Fat 3g | Carbs 26g | Fibre 10g | Protein 6g

Date	Time	Blood glucose level before meal	Blood glucose level 2 hours after meal	After-meal blood glucose on target (y/n)?	Notes, e.g. any changes made to recipe or portion size

BAKED EGGS WITH MUSHROOMS

Serves 4

30g (1oz) unsalted butter
250g (9oz) button mushrooms, thinly sliced, stalks
*   removed (use to make a creamy sauce)*
4 eggs
small bunch of parsley, chopped
sourdough bread, to serve
salt and freshly ground black pepper, to taste

Preheat the oven to 160°C/325°F/gas mark 3.

Add roughly two-thirds of the butter to a frying pan and melt over a medium heat. As soon as the butter starts to froth, add the mushrooms and cook until they have released all their juices and have softened, about 10 minutes. Season with salt and pepper.

Grease 4 small ovenproof dishes with the remaining butter, divide the mushrooms between them and carefully break an egg over each one. Season again with a little salt and bake in the oven for about 10 minutes or until the egg whites have thoroughly set.

Sprinkle lightly with the chopped parsley and serve in the individual dishes with a small piece of sourdough bread to mop up the juices.

Nutrition Facts (per serving)
Calories 141 | Total Fat 11g | Sat Fat 6g | Carbs 3g | Fibre 1g | Protein 8.5g

Simple Breakfasts and Brunches

Date	Time	Blood glucose level before meal	Blood glucose level 2 hours after meal	After-meal blood glucose on target (y/n)?	Notes, e.g. any changes made to recipe or portion size

BLUEBERRY QUINOA BREAKFAST

Quinoa, pronounced 'keen-wa', is a wheat-free alternative to starchy grains. Considered a superior alternative to bulgur wheat, couscous and rice, quinoa is, botanically speaking, a member of the same family as beets, chard and spinach. Quinoa contains all nine essential amino acids, making it a complete protein source. The blueberries give a little freshness to the bowl, and the walnuts add a lovely crunchy texture.

Serves 4
100ml (3½fl oz) water
400ml (14fl oz) full-cream milk
150g (5¼oz) quinoa, rinsed
1 tsp pure vanilla essence
½ tsp ground cinnamon
200g (7oz) blueberries
30g (1oz) walnuts, chopped (optional)

Put the water and milk in a saucepan and bring to the boil. Add the quinoa and simmer over a gentle heat for 15 minutes. Once cooked, strain the quinoa and return it to the pan. Stir in the vanilla essence and cinnamon before dividing the mixture among 4 breakfast bowls.

Top the quinoa with blueberries and walnuts, if you like.

Nutrition Facts (per serving)

Calories 286 | Total Fat 11g | Sat Fat 3g | Carbs 37g | Fibre 4.6g | Protein 10g

Date	Time	Blood glucose level before meal	Blood glucose level 2 hours after meal	After-meal blood glucose on target (y/n)?	Notes, e.g. any changes made to recipe or portion size

BAKED FIGS WITH GOAT'S CHEESE AND BALSAMIC VINEGAR GLAZE

The fruit of the *ficus* tree, figs have a culinary history that goes back to antiquity. Their soft and chewy texture offset by crunchy edible seeds and unctuous sweet taste combines quite brilliantly with goat's cheese. You won't come across this simple yet sophisticated recipe on many British breakfast tables, but it has the ability to transport you to warm Mediterranean climes in one stroke.

Serves 2

4 ripe but firm figs
8 slices Parma ham
75g (2½oz) goat's cheese, chopped into small pieces
2 tbsp extra-virgin olive oil
2 tbsp balsamic vinegar
1 tsp freshly ground black pepper

Preheat the oven to 180°C/350°F/gas mark 4.

Using a sharp knife, cut a cross into the top of each fig and then squeeze the fruit at the bottom. It should open up like a flower.

Stuff each one with a good helping of the goat's cheese and carefully wrap two pieces of Parma ham around the middle. Make sure that you leave the tops exposed so that the melted cheese can ooze out.

Now put the wrapped figs in a baking tin and place in the oven for about 8-10 minutes until the cheese has melted and the ham is nice and crisp.

While the figs are in the oven, put the balsamic vinegar in a small saucepan and reduce until you have something approaching a glaze.

Transfer the baked and still warm figs on to serving plates, drizzle with the olive oil and balsamic vinegar and a sprinkling of black pepper.

Nutritional value per serving
Calories 485 | Total Fat 34g | Sat Fat 13.5g | Carbs 27g | Fibre 3.5g | Protein 19g

Date	Time	Blood glucose level before meal	Blood glucose level 2 hours after meal	After-meal blood glucose on target (y/n)?	Notes, e.g. any changes made to recipe or portion size

WHEAT-FREE PANCAKES WITH GREEK YOGHURT AND FRUIT

These unsweetened pancakes go brilliantly with full-fat Greek-style yoghurt along with fresh fruit and berries. This mixture should make 10 or more pancakes, depending on how big your frying pan is and how many you flip onto the floor!

Serves 4

350g (12½oz) almond flour
1 tbsp flaxseed, lightly crushed in a pestle and mortar
½ tsp bicarbonate of soda
pinch of sea salt
3 eggs
180ml (6½fl oz) unsweetened almond 'milk'
2 tbsp unsalted butter, melted, plus a little extra for frying

Put the flour, flaxseed, bicarbonate of soda and salt in a bowl and mix thoroughly.

In a separate large bowl, whisk the eggs with the milk. Carefully add the melted butter, which should be just warm (you don't want to end up with a scrambled egg mix at this stage). Gradually whisk the flour mix into the egg mix. If it is too dry, add more almond milk, a tablespoon at a time, until you have a smooth, wet pancake batter.

Heat a nugget of butter in a non-stick frying pan and when it is hot add 4 tablespoons of the batter. Swirl it about until it covers the pan and cook for 3 minutes (you should see the edges lift and turn brown). Flip it over (we've all seen chefs tossing pancakes) and cook the other side for 3 minutes before turning out onto a warmed plate.

Nutrition Facts (per serving)
Calories 614 | Total Fat 54g | Sat Fat 8g | Carbs 7g | Fibre 10g | Protein 24g

Date	Time	Blood glucose level before meal	Blood glucose level 2 hours after meal	After-meal blood glucose on target (y/n)?	Notes, e.g. any changes made to recipe or portion size

PEPPER, HAM AND TOMATO OMELETTE

This classic method of cooking omelettes should form part of any home cook's repertoire. This recipe is repeated with mushrooms instead in the lunch section, for which we make no apologies. This protein-rich, well-flavoured omelette will give you a terrific start to your day.

Serves 2

4 eggs
½ tbsp olive oil
2 level tbsp unsalted butter
1 medium red pepper, deseeded and finely diced
2 spring onions, white parts separated from the green,
   finely chopped on the diagonal
30g (1oz) mature Cheddar, grated
100g (3½oz) slices wafer-thin ham, shredded
2 medium-ripe tomatoes, cut into wedges
salt and freshly ground black pepper, to taste

Crack the eggs into a large bowl, add salt and plenty of pepper and beat gently with a fork.

Heat a frying pan (20cm/8in is ideal) and once it is very hot add the olive oil and the butter. Once the butter turns a lovely golden colour (but not brown – if it does, start again!) pour in the eggs, give the pan a good shake to even out the surface of the eggs then leave well alone for 30 seconds before very gently stirring with a soft spatula.

The omelette will start to form in front of your eyes, and when it starts to hold its shape but is still underdone in the middle, tip in the pepper, the white part of the spring onions, the cheese and shredded ham. Carefully lift the edge of the omelette and fold it over the filling to the opposite edge of the pan. Cook for 1–2 minutes more.

Transfer the omelette to a warmed plate and cut it in half. Sprinkle with the green part of the spring onions and the tomato wedges and serve immediately.

Nutrition Facts (per serving)
Calories 429 | Total Fat 32g | Sat Fat 15g | Carbs 10g | Fibre 2.3g | Protein 27g

Date	Time	Blood glucose level before meal	Blood glucose level 2 hours after meal	After-meal blood glucose on target (y/n)?	Notes, e.g. any changes made to recipe or portion size

FERGUS HENDERSON'S KIPPERS

A kipper is a smoked herring and is a veritable king among breakfasts. Fergus Henderson, chef founder of St John restaurant in London's EC1 (www.stjohngroup.uk.com), rightly says that a brace of kippers makes the perfect start to the day.

Serves 1

1 kipper

butter, for cooking

sourdough toast, to serve (optional)

Preheat the oven to 200°C/400°F/gas mark 6.

Put the kipper in a baking dish and top with large lumps of butter. Bake in the oven for 10 minutes.

Eat it with sourdough toast, if you like, and wash it all down with lashings of hot strong breakfast tea.

Nutrition Facts (per 75g of kipper serving)
Calories 357 | Total Fat 34g | Sat Fat 16g | Carbs 0 | Fibre 0g | Protein 15g

Date	Time	Blood glucose level before meal	Blood glucose level 2 hours after meal	After-meal blood glucose on target (y/n)?	Notes, e.g. any changes made to recipe or portion size

LIGHT LUNCHES, SALADS AND SOUPS

CRAB ON AVOCADO WITH CORIANDER-INFUSED OLIVE OIL AND HERB SALAD

Serves 2

Crab has a sweet, intense, succulent flavour and goes brilliantly with coriander and avocado. The flavour of the oil is more intense if it is prepared a day ahead and kept in the fridge. If you like, you can mop up the last bits of oil with a chunk of sourdough bread.

200g (7oz) white crabmeat
2 tbsp full-fat crème fraîche
1 tsp cayenne pepper
1 tbsp coriander, roughly chopped
1 ripe medium avocado
juice of 1 lime
salt and freshly ground pepper, to taste

For the coriander-infused olive oil
1 tsp coriander seeds
1 tsp cumin seeds
1 tsp fennel seeds
150ml (5¼fl oz) virgin olive oil
½ tsp turmeric
small bunch of coriander leaves, washed

For the herb salad
large handful of flat-leaf parsley, leaves only
large handful of tarragon
   large handful of chervil
1 tbsp capers in brine, rinsed and drained
1 shallot, thinly sliced
2 tbsp extra-virgin olive oil, plus extra to serve
1 tbsp red wine vinegar

To make the infused oil, lightly crush the coriander, cumin and fennel seeds in a pestle and mortar. In a heavy-based pan, toast the crushed spices on a medium heat until they are lightly brown and are giving up their oils, about 2–3 minutes. Add the olive oil, stir in the turmeric and set over a very low heat for 30 minutes to allow the flavours to infuse.

Meanwhile, blanch the coriander leaves in a pan of boiling water for 1 minute then refresh in a colander set in iced water. Drain. Remove the oil from the heat, allow to cool for 10 minutes and then strain through a sieve into a bowl. Add the drained coriander and blitz thoroughly with a hand blender. Refrigerate until ready to use.

In a bowl (preferably metal) mix the crab, crème fraîche, cayenne pepper and chopped coriander with plenty of salt and pepper. Peel the avocado carefully, cut it in half and remove the stone. Put the avocado flesh in a bowl and mash thoroughly with the lime juice and season well. Chill in the fridge for at least 30 minutes.

To make the herb salad, simply mix all the herbs, capers and shallot in a bowl. Add the olive oil to the red wine vinegar in a small dish and pour over the salad. Toss through once and chill in the fridge until you are ready to serve.

Place a 9cm (3½inch) ring mould on each plate and carefully spoon half of the avocado into each one. Smooth the surface of the avocado with the back of the spoon and then top with the crabmeat. Remove the moulds, drizzle the coriander oil around and serve immediately with the herb salad and an extra glug of olive oil, if you like.

Nutritional value per serving
Calories 244 | Total Fat 13g | Sat Fat 2g | Carbs 9g | Fibre 5g | Protein 22g

Date	Time	Blood glucose level before meal	Blood glucose level 2 hours after meal	After-meal blood glucose on target (y/n)?	Notes, e.g. any changes made to recipe or portion size

SARDINES WITH A GREEK-STYLE SALAD

Very rich in omega-3 fatty acids, sardines are also extremely tasty and versatile – you can grill, roast, fry and barbecue them to perfection. In fact, it's pretty hard to go wrong with them, so let's all of us eat a lot more of these shimmering and relatively sustainable little fish.

If buying fresh, the usual rules apply – try to buy sardines that have bright eyes and shiny skin with the scales intact and pink flesh with a fine, soft texture. Avoid cloudy eyes that say, 'I am, sadly, not a fish of the quality you would want to eat'. If you are going to prepare the sardines yourself, either cook them whole or you can spend a rather tedious amount of time filleting them. Chefs have people to do this for them; at home cook them whole as life is too short. Save yourself a job and have your fishmonger gut and descale the fish for you.

Serves 4

2 x 135g (4¾oz) cans sardines in olive oil (with or
  without chilli or tomato, as you prefer), drained,
  or 8 whole fresh sardines
olive oil, for cooking
lemon juice, for squeezing over
salt and freshly ground black pepper, to taste
buttered brown bread, to serve

For the salad

> *2 tbsp extra-virgin olive oil*
> *juice of 1 lemon*
> *1 garlic clove, finely chopped*
> *2 tsp chopped oregano (or 1 tsp dried oregano)*
> *½ tsp freshly ground black pepper*
> *4 medium tomatoes, quartered*
> *½ medium cucumber, skinned and cut into bite-sized chunks*
> *160g (5½oz) canned chickpeas (or black-eyed beans), rinsed and drained*
> *75g (2½oz) feta cheese, crumbled*
> *½ medium red onion, thinly sliced*
> *2 tbsp green olives, sliced in half*
> *2 tbsp black olives, sliced in half*

Preheat the oven to 200°C/400°F/gas mark 6.

If you are using fresh sardines, rub the fish with olive oil, salt and pepper and place them in a hot heavy-based pan that has been smeared with olive oil. Canned sardines are already well coated with oil and don't need any more. Cook on a high heat each side for 3–4 minutes until the flesh easily flakes away from the bones. Remove to a warm plate and a drizzle over a little lemon juice. This helps counteract the intense oily flavour the fish can have. Or heat a griddle pan until it is very hot, rub each fish with olive oil and sear the sardines for 1 minute on both sides.

Now lay them in an oiled roasting tin and cook in the oven for 6–8 minutes.

To make the salad, whisk the oil, lemon juice, garlic, oregano and pepper in a large bowl to combine. Add the tomatoes, cucumber, chickpeas (or black-eyed beans), feta cheese, onion and olives. Gently toss to combine everything.

Divide the salad among 4 plates and top each with a couple of sardines. A small piece of well-buttered brown bread to soak up the juices helps things along enormously.

Nutritional value per serving
Calories 393 | Total Fat 23g | Sat Fat 13g | Carbs 19g | Fibre 8g | Protein 34g

Date	Time	Blood glucose level before meal	Blood glucose level 2 hours after meal	After-meal blood glucose on target (y/n)?	Notes, e.g. any changes made to recipe or portion size

WHOLE SARDINES WITH A WARM OLIVE AND BEETROOT SALAD

Home-cooked sardines are a delight when served on an olive-oil-rich, warm autumnal salad. This recipe is based on a quite wonderful dish served at the East Beach Café in Littlehampton, on the south coast. This salad would work just as well with fillets of smoked trout. If you have bought olives that are in jars of brine, set them in a colander and wash them under cold running water then dry with kitchen paper, otherwise they will be too salty.

Serves 4

1 tbsp extra-virgin olive oil, plus extra for the fish
8 whole fresh sardines, gutted and descaled
juice of ½ lemon
1 tsp chopped parsley
sea salt flakes and freshly ground black pepper, to taste
buttered brown bread, to serve

For the salad
2 tbsp green olives, pitted and cut in half
2 tbsp black olives, pitted and cut in half
2 tbsp extra-virgin olive oil
1 tsp finely chopped fresh chervil
1 tsp finely chopped fresh oregano
1 red chilli, sliced
3 medium tomatoes, quartered
2 small cooked beetroot, cut into small dice

First, marinate the olives in olive oil, the herbs and chilli in a bowl covered with cling film for about an hour, or overnight in the fridge.

Heat 1 tablespoon of olive oil in a heavy-based pan but do not allow the oil to smoke. Rub the sardines with olive oil, salt and pepper and pan-fry for 3–4 minutes on each side. Remove the pan from the heat, lift the fish onto a warm plate and sprinkle over the lemon juice. Cover with tin foil and set aside.

Lower the heat. Now add the tomatoes, beetroot and marinated olives along with their herby oil to the same pan and cook everything on a gentle heat until the tomatoes are soft, for 10–15 minutes.

Divide the warm salad among four bowls, tipping over the remaining oil from the pan, season with a little pepper and place 2 sardines on top of dish. Sprinkle over a few sea salt flakes and the parsley and serve immediately with small slices of well-buttered brown bread.

Nutritional value per serving
Calories 627 | Total Fat 38g | Sat Fat 16g | Carbs 6g | Fibre 1.2g | Protein 61g

Date	Time	Blood glucose level before meal	Blood glucose level 2 hours after meal	After-meal blood glucose on target (y/n)?	Notes, e.g. any changes made to recipe or portion size

BROKEN SARDINES WITH AN AVOCADO AND FENNEL SALAD

Serves 4

12 cherry tomatoes, cut in half
½ tsp sea salt
85ml (3fl oz) virgin olive oil
juice of 1 lime
½ medium red onion, roughly chopped
½ medium cucumber, halved lengthwise, peeled, seeds
*   removed and cut into chunks*
1 fennel, roughly chopped
8 radishes, roughly chopped
½ bunch of coriander, washed and chopped
1 ripe avocado, peeled, stoned and flesh chopped
2 x 135g (4¾oz) cans sardines in olive oil, drained
buttered brown bread, to serve
freshly ground black pepper, to taste

Put the tomatoes in a largish bowl and add the sea salt, olive oil and lime juice. Give everything a good stir to mix. Now add the onion, cucumber, fennel and radishes and toss everything to combine.

Finally, add in the chopped avocado and break the sardines into the salad. Season to taste and eat immediately with a piece or two of brown bread.

Nutritional value per serving

Calories 362 | Total Fat 30g | Sat Fat 5g | Carbs 15g | Fibre 7g | Protein 14g

Date	Time	Blood glucose level before meal	Blood glucose level 2 hours after meal	After-meal blood glucose on target (y/n)?	Notes, e.g. any changes made to recipe or portion size

AVOCADO BAKED WITH EGG AND CHORIZO

This makes a perfect brunch or a lovely light early supper.

Serves 2

1 medium ripe avocado

2 large eggs

2 tbsp olive oil

200g (7oz) chorizo sausage, chopped into 1cm (½in) pieces

2 tsp chopped chives (optional)

4 home-made sunflower seed crackers (page 101), to serve

salt and freshly ground black pepper, to taste

Preheat the oven to 180°C/350°F/gas mark 4.

Cut the avocado in half and remove the stone. Now scoop a little extra of the flesh out so the eggs will fit into the avocado. Scrunch up some tin foil in an ovenproof dish so that you can position the avocado halves upright and there is no wobble.

Separate the eggs yolks and whites into two bowls. Spoon the yolks into the scooped-out avocado, then gently add as much egg white as will fit (you will probably have some left over). Season with salt and pepper. Bake in the oven for 15–20 minutes until the white is opaque and the yolk is at your preferred consistency.

Meanwhile, heat the oil in a heavy-based pan and cook the chorizo until nice and crisp. Remove from the pan and drain on kitchen paper.

Put the avocado and the chorizo on a warmed plate and season well with salt and pepper, then scatter with chopped chives (if using). Serve with the sunflower seed crackers on the side.

Nutritional value per serving
Calories 585 | Total Fat 38g | Sat Fat 8g | Carbs 26g | Fibre 6.4g | Protein 38g

Date	Time	Blood glucose level before meal	Blood glucose level 2 hours after meal	After-meal blood glucose on target (y/n)?	Notes, e.g. any changes made to recipe or portion size

SUNFLOWER SEED CRACKERS

Serves 4

*100g (3½oz) shelled sunflower seeds, plus extra for the
topping*
50g (1¾oz) grated Parmesan
2 tbsp cold water
salt and freshly ground black pepper, to taste

Preheat the oven to 160°C/325°F/gas mark 3.

Put the 100g (3½oz) sunflower seeds in a clean coffee
or spice grinder and process until they are reduced to
a reasonably fine powder-like 'flour'. Tip the sunflower
'flour' into a bowl of a food processor and stir through
the Parmesan. Season with a little salt and pepper. Now
add the water, a tablespoon at a time, and pulse with the
processor until the dough is well blended, soft and sticky.

Cover a baking sheet with a piece of greaseproof
paper. Roll the dough out onto the greaseproof paper
then cover with another sheet of greaseproof paper. Roll
the dough again, through the paper, until it is as thin
and even as you can manage – the thinner the better,
but try to avoid tearing holes in the dough. Peel off the
top layer of parchment then use a pizza cutter or a sharp
pointed knife to score the dough into even, square,
cracker shapes. Carefully push whole sunflower seeds
into the batter.

Bake for 25–30 minutes until evenly browned. Peel off
the greaseproof paper and break along the scored lines

while warm. Cool the crackers on a rack. Once cooled, they can be stored in a container with a tight lid for several weeks.

Nutritional value per serving

Calories 183 | Total Fat 15g | Sat Fat 3g | Carbs 5g | Fibre 3g | Protein 9g

Date	Time	Blood glucose level before meal	Blood glucose level 2 hours after meal	After-meal blood glucose on target (y/n)?	Notes, e.g. any changes made to recipe or portion size

KIDNEYS WITH WHITE CABBAGE, GARLIC, PARSLEY AND BUTTER

Relatively cheap, easy to prepare and very nourishing, lamb's kidneys are great for a quick breakfast, handy lunch or light supper. The general reluctance of people to eat offal is a great shame. These tasty morsels when 'devilled' (meaning prepared with a spicy mustard sauce) are one Victorian invention we should all embrace. This particular dish goes swimmingly with a strong cup of tea or, if you are in the mood to spoil yourself, a glass of robust red wine.

We are indebted to our friends at the exemplary London chain of cafés, Fernandez & Wells, who kindly sent us this recipe – it is taken from their magnificent cookbook, *Rustic*.

Serves 2

300g (10½oz) lamb's kidneys
2 level tbsp salted butter
1 tsp finely chopped flat-leaf parsley
4 garlic cloves, finely chopped
300g (10½oz) white cabbage, finely shredded
2 tsp Dijon mustard
sea salt and freshly ground black pepper, to taste

Prepare the kidneys by removing the clear membrane that covers them. Cut the kidneys in half and remove the white (tough and inedible) core with a sharp pair of scissors. Put 1 tablespoon of butter in a largish frying pan and heat until it has melted and is starting to froth. Add the kidneys and cook them gently over a moderate heat for 2–3 minutes on each side until cooked through. Add the parsley and stir to combine. Season to taste. Remove the kidneys from the pan and keep warm.

Put the rest of the butter in the pan and when melted add the garlic and fry gently for 2 minutes. Add the white cabbage, mustard and a pinch of salt, then add a drop of hot water and cook on a very high heat for 5 minutes, stirring all the time, until the cabbage is cooked through. Serve hot, straight from the pan, with the kidneys.

Nutritional value per serving
Calories 292 | Total Fat 17g | Sat Fat 9g | Carbs 8g | Fibre 4.6g | Protein 26g

Date	Time	Blood glucose level before meal	Blood glucose level 2 hours after meal	After-meal blood glucose on target (y/n)?	Notes, e.g. any changes made to recipe or portion size

TOASTED GOAT'S CHEESE WITH AN AVOCADO, PEAR AND WALNUT SALAD

This delightfully simple recipe comes courtesy of Lancastrian cheesemaker and chef extraordinaire, Sean Wilson. Perhaps better known as Martin Platt of *Coronation Street*, nowadays Sean is the proprietor of the award-winning Saddleworth Cheese Company. Their products are well worth seeking out online and at food fairs.

Goat's cheese has its own slightly acidic and pungent flavour, but once you are a fan, you are hooked for life. It toasts as well as any cheese you can buy. Prepare the avocado and pear just before using, or squeeze over the juice of ½ lime to keep their colour.

Serves 2

110g (4oz) tender baby leaf salad
1 medium ripe avocado, peeled, stoned and flesh cut into small chunks
1 large conference pear, cored and cut into small chunks
3 radishes, topped, tailed and sliced very thinly
1 nectarine, sliced very thinly
1 tbsp chopped walnuts
1 tbsp pumpkin seeds
2 x 35g (1¼oz) good-quality goat's cheeses
15g (½oz) baked or toasted wholemeal breadcrumbs
salt and freshly ground black pepper, to taste

For the vinaigrette
3 tbsp walnut oil
1 tbsp sherry vinegar
juice of ½ lemon

Begin by assembling the salad. In two serving bowls place a good handful of the salad leaves and then layer with the avocado and pear. Dot the radish and nectarine slices around the edges of the salad for colour, and finally scatter over the walnuts and half of the pumpkin seeds.

To make the vinaigrette, put the walnut oil, sherry vinegar and lemon juice in a bowl and whisk vigorously to combine. Check the seasoning – a little salt and a good grind of pepper will add a good depth of flavour.

With a sharp knife, carefully remove the top rind from each goat's cheese and then grill the cheeses on a high heat until the top is bubbling and turning brown and the cheese is warmed through. Place the grilled goat's cheese on top of the salad and generously drizzle with the vinaigrette. Finally, scatter the remaining pumpkin seeds and the breadcrumbs over the cheese and serve immediately.

Nutritional value per serving
Calories 552 | Total Fat 48g | Sat Fat 9.5g | Carbs 24g | Fibre 9.8g | Protein 11g

Light Lunches, Salads and Soups

Date	Time	Blood glucose level before meal	Blood glucose level 2 hours after meal	After-meal blood glucose on target (y/n)?	Notes, e.g. any changes made to recipe or portion size

LAMB AND LEEK BROTH

A good Scotch broth should look somewhat unpre-possessing when served, lacking colourful highlights or much in the way of sophistication, but lamb when stewed in its own juices supplies a flavour like no other. You will need a good few hours to arrive at the perfect broth, but on a cold February day, few dishes will hit the spot quite like this. Delicious with a piece or two of brown bread and butter to mop up the juices.

Serves 6

1kg (2lb) lamb (the scrag end of neck or any cheap
   cut), sliced into chunks
200g (7oz) carrots, roughly diced
100g (3½oz) turnip (or swede), roughly diced
1 small white onion, roughly chopped
2 celery sticks, finely chopped
2 leeks, outer layer removed, washed, trimmed and chopped
4 cloves
2 bay leaves
70g (4oz) pearl barley
bunch of parsley, stalks removed and leaves chopped
Worcestershire sauce, to serve (optional)
sea salt and freshly ground black pepper, to taste

Put the lamb in a large casserole dish and cover with cold water. On the hob, bring the water to a very gentle simmer and then, using a large flat spoon, scoop off the scum as it rises to the top. Continue to simmer for 45 minutes, periodically removing any scum that has the temerity to appear.

Preheat the oven to 130°C/250°F/gas mark ½. Now add the carrots, turnip (or swede), onion, celery, leeks, cloves and bay leaves. Bring everything back to a simmer and remove any scum before putting on a tight-fitting lid and transferring the pot to the oven. Cook for at least 1 hour until the lamb is very tender.

With a pair of tongs, remove the lamb pieces to a large plate and allow to cool. Add the pearl barley to the stock, give it a good stir, then return the pot to the hob, bring it back to a gentle simmer and cook for at least 20 minutes.

Once it is cool enough to handle, shred the lamb with your fingers. This is a messy job, but peculiarly enjoyable. Discard any bits of bones and fatty pieces that escaped initial scrutiny, and feel free to chop the lamb pieces with a sharp knife if you want to. Stir the lamb back into the simmering stock and keep it on the hob for another 5–10 minutes until the pearl barley is tender. Adjust the seasoning, being particularly robust with the black pepper.

Serve in individual soup bowls while steaming hot, topped with a generous sprinkling of chopped parsley and a shot of Worcestershire sauce, if you like.

Tip
Lamb has a high fat content and you may find that your broth is a bit too fatty for your tastes, so feel free to

remove some of it, but do leave some as the fat adds a lot of flavour and is nutritionally important. You can soak up excess fat by placing kitchen paper on the top of the stew when you remove the pot from the heat, or let it cool completely, put it in the fridge overnight and the fat can be easily scraped off with a spoon the following day. Actually, there is something to be said for serving this broth the next day – somehow it's even tastier twenty-four hours on.

Nutritional value per serving

Calories 480 | Total Fat 30g | Sat Fat 14g | Carbs 20g | Fibre 5g | Protein 34g

Date	Time	Blood glucose level before meal	Blood glucose level 2 hours after meal	After-meal blood glucose on target (y/n)?	Notes, e.g. any changes made to recipe or portion size

(SORT OF) GERMAN LENTIL SOUP

We have been cooking with lentils for 2,000 years or more. They belong to the same family as beans – legumes – which means they share the same benefits in that they are a rich source of fibre and lean protein.

This recipe can really have no claim on authenticity, and any German citizen worth their culinary salt will be demanding the immediate return of *fetter Speck* – a cured pork fat that positively oozes a taste-rich fat when heated – to replace the butter. If you want to be authentic, track down this fat in a German deli along with the sausages by all means, there's no doubt it does add flavour.

Serves 6

2 level tbsp unsalted butter
250g (8oz) good-quality smoked bacon, cut into lardons
4 garlic cloves, finely chopped
100g (3½oz) swede, peeled and roughly diced
400g (14oz) can plum tomatoes
2 red peppers, deseeded and diced
2 carrots, diced
1 onion, roughly chopped
1 large leek, trimmed, washed and sliced
1 celery stick, finely chopped
1¾ litres (3 pints) water or light chicken stock
100g (3½oz) brown lentils, rinsed and drained
200g (7oz) grilled Frankfurters, sliced

bunch of flat-leaf parsley, stems discarded, leaves
  chopped
salt and freshly ground black pepper, to taste

Heat the butter in a large casserole dish until it is frothing, add the bacon and cook for 4–5 minutes, stirring occasionally, until browned on both sides. Add the garlic and continue to cook for 2–3 minutes until it starts to turn a golden colour. Now add the swede, tomatoes, peppers, carrots, onion, leek and celery. Stir everything to mix and cook for 5 minutes, giving it all an occasional additional stir. Pour in the water or stock and bring to the boil then immediately turn down the heat. Add the lentils and gently simmer for 50–60 minutes with the lid on. When there is 10 minutes to go, add the grilled Frankfurters.

When you are ready to serve, adjust the seasoning carefully and stir in the parsley. Serve piping hot and if you can find any German dark *Brot* (bread) studded with seeds to go with it, so much the better.

Tip
Prepare the lentils according to the instructions on the packet. This will almost certainly involve sorting through and discarding any hardened kernels, grit, etc., washing them in 3–4 changes of clean water and finally soaking them in enough water to cover for at least 30 minutes.

Nutritional value per serving

Calories 486 | Total Fat 32g | Sat Fat 10g | Carbs 19g | Fibre 3g | Protein 25g

Date	Time	Blood glucose level before meal	Blood glucose level 2 hours after meal	After-meal blood glucose on target (y/n)?	Notes, e.g. any changes made to recipe or portion size

TOMATO SOUP

Everybody should make home-made tomato soup and avoid the expensive and less healthy canned varieties. It's so easy to make, keeps in the fridge for a day or two and freezes well. Once you have established your regular recipe you can do all sorts of things with it – add lentils, swap oregano for the basil, forgo the crème fraîche and add a red chilli or two, reduce the amount of stock, blitz the onions and garlic before adding the tomatoes to produce a rich, lumpy, tomato stew, or add a couple of red peppers and sherry vinegar for a Spanish touch.

A word about tomatoes: it has to be said that supermarket varieties in the UK are an endless source of disappointment – the climate doesn't help, but there is little excuse for the largely tasteless, uniform, red squash balls that we are routinely offered. You will be rewarded with a far more flavoursome soup (or salad, for that matter) if you or your friends and neighbours grow your own, or seek out heirloom (sometimes know as heritage) varieties at farmers' markets.

Serves 6

1½kg (3½lb) very ripe (on the squidgy side) tomatoes, skinned (see tip)

3 tbsp virgin olive oil, plus extra to serve

2 tbsp balsamic vinegar

1 large Spanish onion, roughly chopped

4 garlic cloves, roughly chopped

1¾ litres (3 pints) chicken or vegetable stock with a
tablespoon of tomato purée
6–10 basil leaves, torn (or use 1 level tsp of dried, if you
must)
100ml (3½fl oz) crème fraîche, to serve (optional) or
for a really rich finish, add a dollop of double cream
sea salt and freshly ground black pepper, to taste

Line your grill pan with tin foil, turning up the edges
so you have a sort of tin bowl. Lay the tomatoes on the
foil and give them a good coating of using most of the
olive oil, a generous sprinkling of balsamic vinegar and
a grind of black pepper. Place under the grill on a high
heat for 6–10 minutes until the edge of the tomatoes are
blackened. Or you can put them in the oven and roast for
25 minutes at 180°C/350°F/gas mark 4.

In a large heavy-based pan, gently heat the remaining
olive oil before adding the onion. Cook for 10–12
minutes, stirring from time to time so that it softens
without colouring. Add the garlic and cook for another
2–3 minutes. Tip in the grilled tomatoes, stir everything
well and cook for another 2–3 minutes before adding the
stock. Bring to a gentle simmer while giving everything
one more good stir. Put on a tight-fitting lid and cook for
about 25 minutes.

Remove from the heat and allow to cool before adding
the basil and blitzing with a hand-held blender. To get an
absolutely smooth texture you can strain it through a fine
sieve, but there's really no need. You should have a soup

that will coat the back of a spoon and is not too watery. If it is still a bit thin, gently reduce it on a medium heat with the lid off.

Adjust the seasoning to taste and serve with a dollop of crème fraîche or double cream and a few dribbles of olive oil. Scrumptious!

Tip

Some recipes say leave the skins of tomatoes on, but the effort of removing them is worthwhile as it certainly results in a sweeter taste and smoother constituency. Bring a large pan of water to the boil and tip in the tomatoes. After a few minutes you will see the skins on most of the tomatoes split. Tip the tomatoes into a colander and run the cold tap over them for a couple of minutes until they've cooled sufficiently to handle. Now the messy bit... On a clean work surface, peel the skin off each tomato (discard) and quarter each. With your thumb, 'eject' the seeds into a bowl – you want to leave a few in some of the tomatoes as they provide a balancing acidity, but too many seeds and the soup tends to have a noticeably sour taste.

Nutritional value per serving

Calories 185 | Total Fat 7.5g | Sat Fat 4.3g | Carbs 23g | Fibre 4.3g | Protein 8.3g

Light Lunches, Salads and Soups

Date	Time	Blood glucose level before meal	Blood glucose level 2 hours after meal	After-meal blood glucose on target (y/n)?	Notes, e.g. any changes made to recipe or portion size

WATERCRESS AND POTATO SOUP

Vibrant in colour and smooth as velvet, you can serve this refreshing soup either hot with a dollop of crème fraîche or chilled with a drizzle of olive oil on a summer's day.

Serves 4

2 tbsp extra-virgin olive oil, plus more to serve

1 banana shallot (or medium onion), finely chopped

200g (7oz) waxy potatoes (Charlottes, for example), peeled and diced

750ml (1½ pints) vegetable stock

1 tsp vegetable bouillon

400g (14oz) watercress, well washed in cold water

130g (4½oz) baby spinach leaves

sea salt and freshly ground black pepper, to taste

In a large heavy-based pan, gently heat the olive oil then add the shallot and potatoes. Cook for 10–12 minutes, stirring from time to time, so that they soften without colouring.

Pour in the stock and vegetable bouillon and bring to the boil. Now add the watercress and spinach, stir through and as soon as the leaves wilt, remove the pan from the heat.

With a slotted spoon or tongs, carefully remove the leaves and potatoes from the pan and transfer to a food processor. Start the blender and gently add the liquid, a drop at a time, as the leaves are thoroughly blitzed. When you have a very smooth texture return everything to the pan. Adjust the seasoning to taste and reheat gently if you are serving the soup hot and serve with a dollop of crème fraîche, or allow it to cool to room temperature with the lid on before chilling in the fridge and serving with a drizzle of olive oil.

Nutritional value per serving
Calories 154 | Total Fat 9.3g | Sat Fat 2.5g | Carbs 16g | Fibre 4g | Protein 5.6g

Date	Time	Blood glucose level before meal	Blood glucose level 2 hours after meal	After-meal blood glucose on target (y/n)?	Notes, e.g. any changes made to recipe or portion size

CURRIED PARSNIP SOUP

This is the ultimate delicious winter warmer. Add more chilli powder to increase the heat, but try not to swamp the natural flavours of the vegetables. You can swap the parsnips for carrots if you prefer.

Serves 4

1 tsp coriander seeds

1 tsp cumin seeds

½ tsp black peppercorns

¼ tsp turmeric

½ tsp chilli powder or ½ tsp chilli flakes

2 tsp garam masala

2 medium onions, roughly chopped

*2cm (1in) piece of fresh root ginger, peeled and cut into
    3–4 pieces*

3 garlic cloves

2 tbsp olive oil

1 tbsp unsalted butter

2 parsnips, peeled and diced

1½ litres (2½ pints) chicken stock or water

*bunch of fresh coriander, stems removed,
    leaves washed and roughly chopped*

*175g (6oz) Greek-style full-fat yoghurt,
    to serve (optional, but you miss a treat
    without it)*

salt and freshly ground black pepper, to taste

Grind the coriander, cumin and black peppercorns in a pestle and mortar or a spice grinder. Add the turmeric, chilli (powder or flakes) and half of the garam masala to the mix.

Put a quarter of the chopped onions, the ginger and garlic into a small food blender with 1 tablespoon of water and blitz until you have a smooth paste. Tip in the spice mix and blend for another 30 seconds until everything is well mixed. Have a good sniff (it will smell wonderful) and set aside.

Heat the olive oil in a deep heavy-based pan and add the butter. Once the butter has melted add the rest of the onions and cook until translucent, stirring all the time. Now tip in the spiced mix, turn up the heat slightly and cook, stirring, for 5 minutes, but don't let it dry out. Add the parsnips, giving them a good stir so that they are well coated with the spice and onion mix and cook for another 5 minutes or so. Pour in the stock, bring to a gentle simmer, put on a tight-fitting lid and cook on a very low heat for 35–40 minutes. About 15 minutes before the end of the cooking time, add in half of the chopped coriander leaves and the rest of the garam masala. Remove from the heat and allow to cool a little before thoroughly blitzing with a hand-held blender. Once you have a nice smooth consistency and have adjusted the seasoning, you are ready to serve.

Pour into individual serving bowls, dollop a good spoonful of Greek full-fat yoghurt into the middle and sprinkle with the rest of the coriander leaves. It will warm the very cockles of your heart.

Nutritional value per serving
Calories 275 | Total Fat 16g | Sat Fat 7g | Carbs 19g | Fibre 4.4g | Protein 13g

Date	Time	Blood glucose level before meal	Blood glucose level 2 hours after meal	After-meal blood glucose on target (y/n)?	Notes, e.g. any changes made to recipe or portion size

TRADITIONAL TARKA DAL

This is a classic accompaniment in India and is served with most meals. It makes a splendid midday lunch with cauliflower cooked with onion and tomato (page 126).

Serves 4

425ml (15fl oz) water

85g (2oz) red split lentils, rinsed

1 medium onion, quartered

3 garlic cloves, halved

¼ tsp turmeric

1 tsp garam masala

2 tbsp ghee or clarified butter, or use cold-pressed
   rapeseed oil (see tip)

1 medium tomato, chopped

2 tbsp chopped coriander leaves

sea salt and freshly ground black pepper, to taste

Pour the water into a pan and bring it to the boil, add a good teaspoon of salt and tip in the lentils. Bring back to the boil then turn the heat down and gently simmer, uncovered, for 20 minutes. Keep skimming off the froth that will collect on the surface. Partially cover the pan and cook for another 40 minutes until you have a yellowish, soup-like consistency.

Meanwhile, put half of the onion and the garlic into a small food blender with a tablespoon of water and blitz until you have a smooth paste. Add in the turmeric and garam masala and blend for another 30 seconds until everything is well combined.

In a heavy-based frying pan, heat the ghee or butter and add the rest of the onion. Cook until the onion is lightly browned and then add the spiced paste, stir thoroughly and cook for another 5 minutes. Tip into the lentils, adjust the seasoning and top with the chopped tomato and coriander. Serve immediately.

Tip
You can buy clarified butter, but it is really easy to prepare yourself. Put the butter in a heavy-based pan over a very low heat and gently melt it. A white froth will soon appear on the surface, which you should remove with a spoon. Now you will see a clear yellow-tinged layer of fat sitting on top of a milky cloudy layer. Carefully pour the yellow fat into a bowl leaving the milky residue in the pan, which should be discarded.

Clarification removes any impurities; clarified butter keeps for several weeks in the fridge and months in the freezer.

Nutritional value per serving
Calories 158 | Total Fat 7.5g | Sat Fat 0.5g | Carbs 16g | Fibre 4g | Protein 6.2g

Light Lunches, Salads and Soups

Date	Time	Blood glucose level before meal	Blood glucose level 2 hours after meal	After-meal blood glucose on target (y/n)?	Notes, e.g. any changes made to recipe or portion size

CAULIFLOWER WITH ONION AND TOMATO

A great 'goes with anything' vegetable staple that will accompany just about any spiced meat dish. This is adapted from a recipe supplied by a good friend in Delhi.

Serves 4

1 medium cauliflower, outer leaves removed and cut into small florets

1 medium onion, roughly chopped

4 garlic cloves, cut in half

2cm (1in) piece fresh root ginger, peeled and chopped into 2 or 3

1 tsp ground coriander

1 tsp ground cumin

2 tsp lightly crushed black peppercorns (use a pestle and mortar)

½ t tsp turmeric

¼ tsp chilli powder

2 tsp garam masala

3 tbsp ghee or clarified butter, or use cold-pressed rapeseed oil (see tip on p124)

juice of ½ lemon

1 fresh green chilli, deseeded and finely chopped

200g (7oz) can chopped tomatoes with their juice or 400g (14oz) fresh tomatoes, peeled, deseeded and finely chopped

1 tsp salt flakes

Wash the cauliflower florets in salted water, then rinse them under cold running water and drain.

Put half of the onion, half of the garlic and all of the ginger into a small food blender along with a little water and blitz until you have a fine paste. Add the ground coriander, cumin, half of the crushed peppercorns, the turmeric, chilli powder and 1 teaspoon of the garam masala and blitz again until everything is well mixed. You should end up with a marvellous-smelling brownish-coloured paste.

In a deep heavy-based pan (or karahi, if you have one), heat the ghee or butter until it is hot but not smoking. Add the cauliflower and 'stir-fry' for 2–3 minutes until the florets have picked up noticeable brown spots. You may need to do this in batches. Remove from the heat and transfer the cauliflower into a bowl with a slotted spoon or tongs and set aside.

Return the pan to the hob, lower the heat, ensure there is still plenty of fat in the pan and add the remaining onions. Cook for 5–7 minutes until they soften but have not browned. Add the remaining garlic and cook for another 2 minutes. Now add the spice paste and cook for 3–4 minutes, stirring all the time. Don't let it dry out, add a tablespoon of water if it starts to catch. Once the onions are cooked, add a good squeeze of lemon juice, the chopped chilli, tomatoes and the remaining crushed black peppercorns. Stir and cook for 2–3 minutes before returning the cauliflower to the pan. Add 4 tablespoons of water, stir well so that the cauliflower is well coated, then cover and simmer for 7–10 minutes, stirring occasionally to make sure nothing is sticking, until the cauliflower is nicely *al dente.*

Remove the pan from the heat and sprinkle over the remaining garam masala and a good sprinkle of salt. Serve while piping hot.

Nutritional value per serving
Calories 278 | Total Fat 25g | Sat Fat 6g | Carbs 8g | Fibre 3.6g | Protein 10g

Date	Time	Blood glucose level before meal	Blood glucose level 2 hours after meal	After-meal blood glucose on target (y/n)?	Notes, e.g. any changes made to recipe or portion size

VEGETABLE CURRY – AS YOU LIKE IT

There really isn't anything in Indian cuisine that equates to the British meat and two veg, but with a little bit of inventiveness you can easily curry seasonal vegetables. Served with a little dal, you have something you might well find at lunchtime in any household in northern India.

You can substitute the pak choi with cabbage, carrots or pretty much any vegetable you like, but adjust the cooking times accordingly.

Serves 4

2 medium onions, roughly chopped

3 garlic cloves

2 tbsp ghee or clarified butter, or cold-pressed rapeseed oil (see page 124)

1 tsp cumin seeds

4 cloves

6 black peppercorns

1 green chilli, deseeded and sliced

1 tsp salt

200g (7oz) cauliflower, cut into small florets

200g pak choi, washed, leaves and stems separated and both cut into strips

200g (7oz) tomatoes, chopped

85g (3oz) fresh or frozen peas (if frozen, defrost first)

Put a quarter of the chopped onions and all the garlic cloves into a small food blender with 1 tablespoon of water and blitz until you have a smooth paste.

Heat a deep heavy-based pan (or karahi) and when piping hot add the cumin seeds, cloves and peppercorns. Cook until the spices release their aromatic oils (2–3 minutes) and then add the ghee or butter to the pan and reduce the heat. Add the remaining onions and cook on a gentle heat for 5–10 minutes until it turns a lovely golden brown.

Now add the onion and garlic paste to the pan along with the sliced chilli and the salt. Stir through and cook for a couple of minutes or so. Add the cauliflower and pak choi stems and cook for 3–4 minutes. Add the tomatoes, making sure you include their juice, and simmer for 10 minutes or until the vegetables are *al dente*. If the pan starts to dry out, add a tablespoon of water. Finally, add the pak choi leaves and the peas and cook for another 3 minutes.

Nutritional value per serving

Calories 147 | Total Fat 7.4g | Sat Fat 0.5g | Carbs 16g | Fibre 4.7g | Protein 4g

Date	Time	Blood glucose level before meal	Blood glucose level 2 hours after meal	After-meal blood glucose on target (y/n)?	Notes, e.g. any changes made to recipe or portion size

SALAMI WITH CELERIAC HASH BROWNS

Serves 4

1 tbsp extra-virgin olive oil, plus extra for frying
150g (5¼oz) salami, thickly sliced
600g (21oz) celeriac, peeled and grated
4 large eggs
3 tbsp butter
1 small aubergine, trimmed and sliced horizontally
2 medium tomatoes, sliced
salt and freshly ground black pepper, to taste

Heat 1 tablespoon of olive oil in a heavy-based deep-sided frying pan then add the salami. Fry, stirring all the time, until it is golden brown on both sides – this should take 10–12 minutes. Remove the salami from the frying pan and set aside.

Put the celeriac into a mixing bowl, crack in 3 of the eggs and give it a careful stir to combine – the mixture should be able to hold its shape in a spoon. Shape the grated celeriac into patties, place on a sheet of greaseproof paper and sprinkle with salt.

Melt the butter in a frying pan over a medium heat, carefully place the patties in the pan and cook for 2–3 minutes on one side until well browned, then flip over and brown the other side.

Meanwhile, beat the remaining egg in a bowl and dip in the aubergine slices. In a second pan, fry the aubergines in olive oil until they are a golden brown on each side.

Divide up the salami, aubergines and celery hash browns among 4 plates and serve with the sliced tomatoes.

Nutritional value per serving
Calories 388 | Total Fat 30g | Sat Fat 12g | Carbs 18.3g | Fibre 4g | Protein 14g

Date	Time	Blood glucose level before meal	Blood glucose level 2 hours after meal	After-meal blood glucose on target (y/n)?	Notes, e.g. any changes made to recipe or portion size

BLACK AND KIDNEY BEAN SOUP

Serves 6

2 tbsp olive oil
1 tbsp unsalted butter
1 Spanish onion, chopped
3 garlic cloves, finely chopped
1 celery stick, finely chopped
1 medium carrot, finely chopped
2 tsp oregano, chopped (or 1 tsp dried)
1½ litres (2½ pints) chicken or vegetable stock
400g (14oz) can black beans, rinsed and drained
200g (7oz) can red kidney beans, rinsed and drained
1 tsp chopped parsley
slices of sourdough, to serve
sea salt and freshly ground black pepper, to taste

In a heavy-based pan heat the olive oil and butter on a medium heat and when the butter has melted and started to froth, cook the onion for 5–7 minutes until it has softened and is just on the point of turning brown. Add the garlic and cook for another 2 minutes. Now add the vegetables and oregano, stir everything to mix and cook for another 3 minutes. Pour in the stock and half of all the beans. Cover and cook for 20 minutes or until the vegetables are tender.

Remove the pan from the heat and cool for 10 minutes before blitzing with a hand-held blender. Carefully adjust the seasoning to taste, add the remaining beans and reheat when you are ready to serve. Sprinkle with the chopped parsley and have a small slice of sourdough bread to hand to mop up the soup.

Nutritional value per serving

Calories 154 | Total Fat 7.5g | Sat Fat 3g | Carbs 21g | Fibre 6g | Protein 6g

Date	Time	Blood glucose level before meal	Blood glucose level 2 hours after meal	After-meal blood glucose on target (y/n)?	Notes, e.g. any changes made to recipe or portion size

CHICKEN AND VEGETABLE SOUP

Serves 6

For the stock

1.3kg (2¾lbs) chicken

2 celery sticks, roughly chopped

1 onion, roughly chopped

1 medium carrot, roughly chopped

1 tsp chopped rosemary

1 tsp chopped thyme

2 bay leaves

6 black peppercorns

For the soup base

2 tbsp olive oil

1 tbsp unsalted butter

1 medium onion, peeled and quartered

2 garlic cloves, finely chopped

2 medium carrots, peeled and finely chopped

2 celery sticks, finely chopped

1 leek, washed and neatly chopped

200g (7oz) Savoy cabbage or cavolo nero, core removed,
*   leaves finely shredded*

1 tbsp grated Parmesan

juice of ½ lemon

salt and freshly ground black pepper, to taste

Place the chicken in a large pan with the celery, onion and carrot and cover with cold water. Wrap the chopped herbs, bay leaves and peppercorns in a sachet of muslin, tie it off and add to the water (or you can use a shop-bought bouquet garni). Bring the stock to the boil, lower the heat and simmer for 45 minutes with the lid on until the chicken meat easily pulls away from the bone. You will need to skim off the scum (and some of the fat) that will rise to the surface from time to time during cooking.

Remove the cooked chicken from the stock and put it on a large plate. Once it is cool enough to handle, remove and discard the skin, then pull the meat from the carcass. Messy, but somehow deeply satisfying.

Skim as much of the fat from the surface of the stock as you can with a spoon, then return the chicken carcass to the pan and simmer for another hour or so with the lid on. The longer you simmer, the better will be the final flavour.

To prepare the base of the soup, begin by heating the olive oil and butter in a deep heavy-based pan. Once the butter starts to froth, add the onion and cook for 5–7 minutes until it starts to soften. Add the garlic and cook for 3 minutes. Stir in the carrots, celery and leek and cook for 3–4 minutes, stirring all the time.

Now carefully strain the stock through a fine sieve into a bowl and discard all the solids. Ideally strain again through muslin, but you might think life is too short… Give the pot a good wipe around with damp kitchen paper to remove any scum or fat, then pour in the strained stock and add the cooked vegetables, 325g (12oz) of the shredded chicken meat, the cabbage or cavolo nero and 1 tablespoon of

Parmesan. Return to the heat for 15 minutes until the vegetables are soft. When you are ready to serve, adjust the seasoning to taste and give it a good squirt of lemon juice to buck it up.

Tip

You will have plenty of chicken meat left over for all manner of cold chicken dishes, such as a Caesar Salad (see page 138).

Nutritional value per serving

Calories 526 | Total Fat 34g | Sat Fat 12g | Carbs 14g | Fibre 4g | Protein 43.3g

Date	Time	Blood glucose level before meal	Blood glucose level 2 hours after meal	After-meal blood glucose on target (y/n)?	Notes, e.g. any changes made to recipe or portion size

CAESAR SALAD

Perhaps the best way to use up leftover chicken is to whip up this most famous of salads. Make no mistake, the mark of a great Caesar salad lies in the quality and quantity of the dressing. Everything else is merely the supporting cast.

While the romaine lettuce is compulsory, there is nothing that says you can't add additional salad items such as spring onions and tomatoes if that's what you fancy. Of course, a 'traditional' Caesar salad features a liberal dose of croutons, something we have removed from our recipe. (If you're ordering this in a restaurant, ask them to 'hold the croutons' and to instead add more salad leaves and a few bits of crispy bacon for extra texture.)

Serves 6

3 romaine hearts (the inner part of a romaine lettuce),
    leaves separated
300g (10½oz) cooked chicken, chopped into bite-sized pieces
200g (7oz) Parmesan

For the dressing:
6 anchovy fillets in olive oil, drained
1 garlic clove
2 large egg yolks
½ tsp Dijon mustard
juice ½ lemon (approx. 2 tbsp)
2 tbsp extra-virgin olive oil
1 tbsp vegetable oil

3 tbsp grated Parmesan
salt and freshly ground black pepper, to serve

First make the dressing. Chop together the anchovy fillets, garlic and a pinch of salt, then transfer to a bowl. Whisk in the egg yolks then add the mustard and the lemon juice. Now carefully (and very gradually) whisk in the olive oil and the vegetable oil until you have a thick, glossy-looking dressing. Finish by folding in the Parmesan, adjust the seasoning and add more lemon juice if you think it needs it. Put the dressing in the fridge until you are ready to assemble the salad.

To assemble the salad, put the romaine lettuce leaves in a large serving bowl, pour over the dressing and use your hands to make sure they are well and truly coated. Add the chicken and, with a vegetable peeler, shave over a modest amount of Parmesan.

Nutritional value per serving
Calories 234 | Total Fat 15.8g | Sat Fat 7g | Carbs 4.2g | Fibre 0.8g | Protein 21.5g

Date	Time	Blood glucose level before meal	Blood glucose level 2 hours after meal	After-meal blood glucose on target (y/n)?	Notes, e.g. any changes made to recipe or portion size

MUSHROOM SOUP

'*Mushrooms have many helpful nutrients, including beta glucans for immune enhancement, ergothioneines for antioxidative potentiation, nerve growth stimulators for helping brain function, and antimicrobial compounds for limiting viruses.*'

PAUL STAMETS (mycologist and advocate for the medicinal benefits of mushrooms)

With their naturally intense, earthy taste, mushrooms are the key ingredients in this classic soup, which supplies a load of creamy comfort and sustenance on a wintery day.

Serves 6
100g (3½oz) dried porcini mushrooms (fresh would be even better)
3 tbsp olive oil
1 level tbsp unsalted butter
1 medium onion, chopped
3 garlic cloves, finely chopped
200g (7oz) Portobello mushrooms, roughly sliced
200g (7oz) chestnut mushrooms, roughly sliced
2 tbsp finely chopped thyme
2 litres (3 pints) vegetable or chicken stock
300ml (10½fl oz) double cream
juice of ½ lemon

1 tbsp chopped parsley, to serve

sea salt and freshly ground black pepper, to taste

Soak the dried porcini mushrooms in hot water for 30 minutes.

Heat 1 tablespoon of olive oil and the butter to a heavy-based pan. Once the butter is frothing, add the onion and cook on a gentle heat until it is translucent, about 5–7 minutes. Add the garlic and cook for another 3 minutes. Put the porcini along with their soaking water and the other chopped mushrooms into the pan and cover with the remaining olive oil, give everything a good stir and cook for a further 10 minutes until the mushrooms release their juices. Add the thyme and a really good grind of black pepper, stir once more and pour in the stock. Cover and cook on a gentle heat for 20 minutes.

Remove from the heat and allow to cool for 5 minutes or so before blitzing with a hand-held blender until you have a lovely silky consistency. Now add the cream, stir, and adjust the seasoning to taste. Finally, add just enough lemon juice to pep it up. Serve with a sprinkling of chopped parsley.

Nutritional value per serving
Calories 359 | Total Fat 27g | Sat Fat 8g | Carbs 24g | Fibre 9g | Protein 10g

Reverse Your Diabetes Diet

Date	Time	Blood glucose level before meal	Blood glucose level 2 hours after meal	After-meal blood glucose on target (y/n)?	Notes, e.g. any changes made to recipe or portion size

OMELETTE WITH GIROLLE MUSHROOMS

Just about everyone ought to make omelettes a regular feature of their diet. Fresh eggs lightly cooked with mushrooms and a little garlic simply can't be bettered. Of course, every chef worth their salt claims to have their own way of making the perfect omelette, but this recipe is a French classic – and has stood the test of time.

Serves 2

4 large eggs

1½ tbsp olive oil

100g (3½oz) girolle mushrooms (or any other wild variety such as ceps or morels), trimmed and wiped over with a damp cloth

1 tbsp chopped parsley

1 small garlic clove, finely chopped

2 tbsp unsalted butter

salt and freshly ground black pepper, to taste

Crack the eggs into a bowl, add salt and pepper and beat gently with a fork.

In a frying pan (20cm/(8in is ideal) heat 1 tablespoon of the olive oil and cook the mushrooms, parsley and garlic for 3–4 minutes – don't let the garlic brown. Season with a little salt and pepper and set aside.

Give the pan a wipe with kitchen paper and return to the heat. Once it is very hot, add the remaining ½ tablespoon of olive oil with the butter. Once the butter turns a lovely golden colour (but not brown – if it goes too far, start again!), pour in the eggs, give the pan a good shake to even out the surface of the omelette and leave well alone for 30 seconds before very gently stirring with a soft spatula.

The omelette will start to form in front of your eyes and when it starts to hold its shape but is still underdone in the middle, tip in the mushrooms. Carefully lift the edge of the omelette and fold it over the mushrooms to the opposite edge of the pan. Cook for 1 more minute.

Now carefully transfer onto a warmed plate and cut it in half to serve.

Nutritional value per serving

Calories 345 | Total Fat 31.5g | Sat Fat 11.7g | Carbs 2.4g | Fibre 1.5g | Protein 14.5g

Date	Time	Blood glucose level before meal	Blood glucose level 2 hours after meal	After-meal blood glucose on target (y/n)?	Notes, e.g. any changes made to recipe or portion size

SALADE NIÇOISE

Ooh la la! Is there a more divisive dish? The usually unpalatable British version, with a pile of cold wet potato and poor-quality canned tuna lumped on top, is pretty far removed from its sunny south-of-France progenitor. This recipe makes no claims for Nice in the Provence-Alpes-Côte d'Azur authenticity, but it is a fresh-tasting chilled summer salad that is great for sharing with friends, especially when eaten *al fresco*.

Serves 2

2 large eggs
50g (1¾oz) fresh broad beans (when in season) or 50g (1¾oz) French beans, trimmed
4 very ripe large tomatoes
¼ cucumber, peeled, quartered, deseeded and cut into chunks
2 spring onions, finely chopped on the diagonal
handful of torn lettuce leaves
½ red pepper, deseeded and thinly sliced
50g (1¾oz) small pitted black olives
1 tbsp capers, rinsed under cold water and drained on kitchen paper
6 anchovies in olive oil, cut into slivers
few basil leaves, roughly torn

For the dressing
50g (1¾oz) pitted black olives
5 anchovies in olive oil, drained
1 garlic clove
juice of ½ lemon
4 tbsp olive oil
1 tbsp balsamic vinegar
salt and freshly ground black pepper, to taste

Have two bowls of water with ice cubes standing by. Put the eggs in a pan of cold water and bring to the boil. Simmer for 7–8 minutes then drop them into one of the bowls of iced water to stop them cooking.

Cook either the broad beans or the French beans in a pan of salted boiling water for 5 minutes or until tender. Refresh in the second bowl of iced water.

Bring a pan of water to the boil and add the tomatoes. You will see the skins start to split. Remove the tomatoes with a slotted spoon to a colander and put under cold running water. Once cool enough to handle, remove the skin, chop into quarters and deseed.

To make the dressing: Make a paste of the olives, anchovies and garlic in a pestle and mortar. Transfer to a bowl and add the lemon juice, olive oil and balsamic vinegar. Season with a grind of black pepper, give everything a good stir and set aside.

To assemble the salad, gently toss the beans, cucumber, spring onions, lettuce, red pepper and tomatoes together.

Add a good slug of the dressing and mix well. Tip onto a large oval serving plate.

Drain and peel the eggs; quarter with a sharp knife and place on the top of the salad. Scatter over the olives, capers, anchovies and basil leaves. Finish by spooning over the remaining dressing and serve immediately.

Tip

If you insist on using tuna then forgo the anchovies, they simply overwhelm the light taste of the fish. To reduce the carbohydrate content of this dish don't include the broad beans.

Nutritional value per serving

Calories 625 | Total Fat 43g | Sat Fat 6g | Carbs 40g | Fibre 10g | Protein 22.4g

Date	Time	Blood glucose level before meal	Blood glucose level 2 hours after meal	After-meal blood glucose on target (y/n)?	Notes, e.g. any changes made to recipe or portion size

AN ITALIAN TUNA SALAD

Having dismissed tuna so peremptorily in the previous recipe, here it is fully reinstated. The recipe calls for tinned tuna and it is worth stating the obvious – the better the quality of the tuna, the nicer the salad will be. Tuna fillets from the venerated Spanish family (and brand) Ortiz are well worth seeking out.

Serves 4

250g (9oz) canned cannellini beans, rinsed and drained

handful of rocket leaves

1 radicchio (Italian chicory), leaves torn

1 red pepper, deseeded and cut into narrow strips

2 ripe medium tomatoes, quartered

1 celery stick, washed, trimmed and cut into thin batons

1 fennel bulb, washed, trimmed (remove the green tops and the shoots and root) and thinly sliced

220g (7¾oz) canned tuna in olive oil, drained and flaked

50g (1¾oz) pitted black olives

4 tbsp extra-virgin olive oil

¼ tsp dried oregano

celery salt and freshly ground black pepper, to taste

brown bread and butter, to serve

In a large bowl toss together the beans, rocket, radicchio, pepper, tomatoes, celery and fennel. Combine the tuna and olives and add to the salad bowl.

In a small bowl mix the olive oil with the oregano and a pinch each of celery salt and pepper. Pour over the salad, give everything a good stir and serve immediately with a small piece of brown bread and butter.

Nutritional value per serving

Calories 331 | Total Fat 20g | Sat Fat 3g | Carbs 20g | Fibre 5g | Protein 20g

Date	Time	Blood glucose level before meal	Blood glucose level 2 hours after meal	After-meal blood glucose on target (y/n)?	Notes, e.g. any changes made to recipe or portion size

AVOCADO AND BEAN SALAD

*'People who put avocados in the fridge are basically saying,
I want to eventually experience something less amazing.'*
GREGOR COLLINS

The avocado is a large berry that contains a single seed
(bet you didn't know that) and is really easy to prepare.
To stop it discolouring while you prepare the other
elements of the recipe, put the flesh in a bowl and sprinkle
it generously with citrus juice, in this case that of a lime.

Serves 4
*400g (14oz) can black (or kidney) beans, drained and
rinsed*
2 large ripe tomatoes, cut into wedges
*½ medium red onion, thinly sliced (use a mandolin if
you have one)*
6 spring onions, chopped on the diagonal
1 whole red chilli, deseeded and finely chopped
*bunch of coriander, stalks removed and the leaves
coarsely chopped*
*1 medium-sized ripe avocado, peeled, stoned and
flesh cut into chunks and sprinkled with the juice
of ½ lime (see tip)*

For the dressing:
grated zest and juice of ½ lime
2 tbsp extra-virgin olive oil
½ tsp organic cider vinegar
salt and freshly ground black pepper, to taste

Put all the ingredients for the salad, except the avocado, into a large bowl and toss thoroughly to mix. Make the dressing by mixing the ingredients in a small bowl and add seasoning to taste. Add the avocado to the salad bowl (along with the lime juice it has been sitting in), give everything a gentle stir and pour over the dressing.

This salad goes particularly well with the chilli con carne on page 169.

Tip
To prepare the avocado, take a sharp knife and run it down vertically from the top to the bottom. You should be able to feel the blade pressing against the stone. Roll the avocado in your hand and cut down the other side. Now gently twist the two halves in opposite directions and you should end up with the two pieces, one in each hand. Use a teaspoon to remove the stone. The skin should easily pull away from the flesh. Finally, cut the flesh into neat 1cm (½in) dice. Put in a bowl and squeeze over the lime juice.

Nutritional value per serving
Calories 224 | Total Fat 14g | Sat Fat 2.3g | Carbs 22g | Fibre 9g | Protein 7g

Reverse Your Diabetes Diet

Date	Time	Blood glucose level before meal	Blood glucose level 2 hours after meal	After-meal blood glucose on target (y/n)?	Notes, e.g. any changes made to recipe or portion size

SMOKED MACKEREL SALAD

A little side helping of either horseradish sauce of wasabi paste adds a certain piquancy if you like that sort of thing.

Serves 4

6 eggs

480g (17oz) smoked mackerel with crushed peppercorns

250g (9oz) roasted red peppers in olive oil
(from a deli or make your own, see tip)

300g (10½oz) green beans, blanched in boiling water
for 3–4 minutes, refreshed in ice water and chopped

100g (3½oz) pitted black olives

100g (3½oz) cherry tomatoes, halved

1 romaine lettuce heart, sliced

4 tbsp olive oil

juice of 1 lime

Start by preparing the eggs. Place in a pan of cold water, bring it to the boil and cook for 7–8 minutes. Refresh the eggs in a bowl of iced water until completely cooled.

Put the smoked mackerel in a bowl and break up with the back of a fork into bite-sized chunks.

Drain the peppers on a few layers of kitchen paper and mix in with the mackerel. Peel the eggs, slice and add into the mackerel along with the beans, olives and tomatoes. Toss everything so that it's well mixed.

Divide the lettuce among 4 plates and place a portion of the mackerel salad on top. Combine the olive oil and lime juice and drizzle over the salad.

Tip
To make your own peppers in oil, cut in half and deseed 2 red peppers, then grill or sear them in a griddle pan until the skin is blackened. Cool, slice into strips and set in a bowl and cover with extra-virgin olive oil.

Nutritional value per serving
Calories 770 | Total Fat 63g | Sat Fat 21g | Carbs 18g | Fibre 5g | Protein 37g

Date	Time	Blood glucose level before meal	Blood glucose level 2 hours after meal	After-meal blood glucose on target (y/n)?	Notes, e.g. any changes made to recipe or portion size

MAIN MEALS

CAPONATA

This is a traditional vegetable- and tomato-based stew from Sicily that has a wonderful sweet and sour taste. It can be eaten hot or cold and either on its own or as a side dish.

Serves 4

1kg (2lbs) tomatoes, peeled, deseeded and chopped, or 2 x
*   450g (14oz) cans chopped tomatoes in their juice*
120ml (4¼fl oz) olive oil
1 medium onion, chopped
1 tbsp white wine vinegar
4 aubergines, diced into 1cm (½in) cubes, well salted
*   and left to drain in a colander for 1 hour*
1 head of celery, sliced
125g (4½oz) green olives, pitted and coarsely chopped
1 tbsp capers, well rinsed

25g (1oz) anchovy fillets, well rinsed in cold water if
salted (or drain on kitchen paper if in oil)
1 tbsp chopped flat-leaf parsley, to serve
salt and freshly ground black pepper

Begin by making the tomato sauce. If using fresh tomatoes, skin them by immersing them in boiling water for twenty seconds or so until the skin starts to split, transfer to a colander and cool under cold running water. The skin should be easy to peel away. Quarter each tomato and scoop out and discard the inner core and seeds. This will lessen the acidity of the finished dish.

Gently heat 1 tablespoon of olive oil in a deep saucepan, add the onion, soften for 5 minutes then add the tomatoes. Allow to cook for a few minutes then add the white wine vinegar and pepper. Simmer on a low heat until you have a dark, well-reduced sauce.

While the tomato sauce is cooking, wash the salt from the aubergine cubes under running water and pat dry on kitchen paper. Fry the aubergine and the celery in a few tablespoons of olive oil in a non-stick frying pan. Add the fried vegetables to the tomato sauce and cook for 30 minutes, stirring from time to time. Add a drop of water to the pan if it starts to get too dry.

Add the olives, capers and anchovies and cook for a further 15 minutes. Remove the pan from the heat and carefully check and adjust the seasoning to taste. Stir in the chopped parsley and serve.

Nutrition Facts (per serving)

Calories 372 | Total Fat 32g | Sat Fat 4g | Carbs 15g | Fibre 7g | Protein 5g

Date	Time	Blood glucose level before meal	Blood glucose level 2 hours after meal	After-meal blood glucose on target (y/n)?	Notes, e.g. any changes made to recipe or portion size

MOUSSAKA

Moussaka is that most famous of Greek dishes made from layers of aubergines and a meat-based sauce. The early history of moussaka is still much debated, but it is thought that it originated when Arabs first introduced the Greeks to aubergines, and there is a thirteenth-century Arabic recipe that certainly resembles it. The Arabs, on the other hand, think the dish is entirely of Greek origin. But then again, early recipes for the moussaka are found in Turkey, which just goes to show that you can't keep the rumour of a great recipe quiet.

Serves 6

2 tbsp good quality extra-virgin cold-pressed
*   rapeseed oil*
500g (1lb) lamb mince
½ tsp dry oregano
1 tsp ground cinnamon
2 tbsp tomato purée
1 glass red wine
1 large onion, sliced
150ml (5½fl oz) extra-virgin olive oil
2 garlic cloves, finely chopped
500g (1lb) skinned and deseeded tomatoes or 400g
*   (14oz) can of chopped tomatoes*
4 small aubergines, cut into slices 1cm (½in) thick and
*   salted (see tip)*
salt and freshly ground black pepper, to taste

For the cream sauce:
75g (3oz) unsalted butter
75g (3oz) plain flour
500ml (1 pint) full-fat milk
55g (2oz) kefalotiri cheese, grated (or use a well-
  flavoured Cheddar)
freshly grated nutmeg
2 large eggs

Preheat the oven to 180°C/350°F/gas mark 4.

Heat the rapeseed oil on a high heat in a frying pan and brown the meat all over – you will need to stir it constantly to break up any lumps and to avoid it catching. Remove from the heat and set aside in a warm place.

In a bowl or measuring jug, mix the oregano, cinnamon, tomato purée, wine and a twist of black pepper.

Fry the onions in some of the olive oil on a gentle heat for 5 minutes until soft then add the garlic and stir through. Cook for 3 more minutes, but do not let the garlic take on colour otherwise it will start to taste unpleasantly bitter. Add the tomatoes, stir through and cook for 5 minutes. Return the meat to the pan and stir so everything is well mixed. Now tip in the spice and wine mix, stir through and simmer gently for 20 minutes or so. Check for seasoning, but be careful with the salt as the final dish will have a salty cheese sauce on top.

Now fry the aubergine. Make sure the pieces are dry before placing them in olive oil in a heavy-based frying pan. Fry on both sides to a golden brown colour and then place them on kitchen paper to drain. Aubergine seems to soak up inordinate amounts of oil so letting them rest on kitchen paper as you go is not a bad idea.

To make the sauce, gently melt the butter in a good-sized saucepan (preferably one with a solid base so that nothing catches during the cooking process). Now add the flour through a sieve, stirring all the time. Once you have added all the flour and cooked it for a few minutes you will have a light golden-coloured roux.

Remove the pan from the heat. Slowly add the milk while whisking constantly with a hand whisk to remove any lumps. Keep adding the milk (at first the milk seems to actually thicken the roux rather than dilute it, but don't worry, keep going) whisking all the while. You should have a thick sauce that easily coats the back of a spoon. Return to the heat and stir in the grated cheese. On a gentle heat, the cheese should melt and be incorporated into the sauce quite easily. If it isn't melting, turn the heat up a little. Finally, season with salt, pepper and grated nutmeg. Remove from the heat and set aside to cool. When cool, gently whisk the two eggs in a bowl then whisk them into the sauce.

To assemble the dish, spread a layer of the meat sauce on the bottom of a deep ovenproof dish (a lasagne dish is ideal) then cover with a layer of aubergine. Continue with alternate layers until you finish with a layer of aubergine. Pour the cream sauce over the top and spread it out so it forms a nice even layer. Bake, uncovered, for about

45 minutes or until the topping is fluffy and a lovely golden brown colour. Serve immediately.

Tip

To prepare aubergines, place them on kitchen paper on a plate and sprinkle with salt, building up layers so that the salted aubergines lie flat. Put a plate on top and weigh down with a couple of heavy saucepans so that the bitter-tasting juice of the aubergines is squeezed out. After 45 minutes tip the aubergines into a colander and wash well under cold running water. Pat dry with kitchen paper.

Nutritional value per serving

Calories 546 | Total Fat 36.6g | Sat Fat 16g | Carbs 24g | Fibre 4g | Protein 24g

Date	Time	Blood glucose level before meal	Blood glucose level 2 hours after meal	After-meal blood glucose on target (y/n)?	Notes, e.g. any changes made to recipe or portion size

RATATOUILLE

This is a classic French stew. The word ratatouille is apparently derived from Latin and means something along the lines of stir and crush. It's a dish that can be made well in advance and eaten either hot or cold, on its own or as an accompaniment to meat, especially lamb.

Serves 4

3 small aubergines

3 medium courgettes

2 medium onions, sliced

100ml (3½fl oz) extra-virgin olive oil

2 garlic cloves, finely chopped

1 red pepper, deseeded and cut into strips

1 green pepper, deseeded and cut into strips

500g (1lb) tomatoes, skinned and deseeded or 400g
   (14oz) can of chopped tomatoes

1 tbsp red wine vinegar

½ tsp coriander seeds, crushed

handful of fresh basil leaves, torn

salt and freshly ground black pepper, to taste

Cut the unpeeled aubergines and courgettes into 1cm (½ in) roundels and place in a colander. Sprinkle liberally with salt and leave to drain for at least 1 hour. Rinse thoroughly under cold running water and dry on kitchen paper.

In a large heavy-based pan, fry the onions in the olive oil on a gentle heat until they soften, but do not allow to brown – about 5–7 minutes. Stir in the garlic and cook for a further 3 minutes, then add the aubergines and peppers. Cover and simmer gently for 20 minutes.

Add the courgettes and tomatoes, season with salt and pepper and add the red wine vinegar.

Cook, uncovered, for 50 minutes until most of the moisture has evaporated from the pan, stirring vigorously from time to time. You don't want the vegetables to break down into a mush; you want an almost sticky, sauce-like consistency. Towards the end, add the crushed coriander seeds and check the seasoning.

Serve either hot or cold sprinkled with torn basil leaves.

Nutritional value per serving

Calories 303 | Total Fat 24g | Sat Fat 4g | Carbs 19g | Fibre 6.5g | Protein 5g

Date	Time	Blood glucose level before meal	Blood glucose level 2 hours after meal	After-meal blood glucose on target (y/n)?	Notes, e.g. any changes made to recipe or portion size

BROCCOLI AND CHICKEN GRATIN

Broccoli was first introduced to England by the Italians some time in the early eighteenth century. Gratins can be unctuous and satisfying; you can vary the quantities of chicken and broccoli so that you do not overwhelm the taste of the meat with the strong-tasting vegetable – or with too much cheese in the sauce for that matter. You can use Calabrese or purple sprouting broccoli for this dish.

Serves 4

*½ free-range roasted chicken, meat pulled off and
    shredded (use the bones for stock)*
500g (1lb) trimmed broccoli broken into small florets
500ml (¾ pint) chicken stock
*1 tsp dried tarragon or a small handful of fresh
    tarragon leaves, torn*
85ml (3fl oz) dry white wine
150ml (5½fl oz) double cream
grated nutmeg, to taste
2 tbsp grated Parmesan
55g (2oz) unsalted butter, plus extra for greasing
55g (2oz) ground almonds

For the béchamel sauce:
75g (3oz) unsalted butter
75g (3oz) plain flour

500ml (1 pint) whole milk
50g (2oz) Cheddar cheese, grated
grated nutmeg, salt and freshly ground black pepper,
to taste

Preheat the oven to 180°C/350°F/gas mark 4.

Start by preparing the béchamel sauce. Gently melt the butter in a good-sized pan, then add the flour, stirring all the time. Once you have added all the flour and cooked it for a few minutes to avoid the unpalatable taste of uncooked flour, you will have a light golden-coloured roux.

Remove the pan from the heat. Slowly add the milk while whisking constantly with a hand whisk to remove any lumps. Keep adding the milk (at first the milk seems to actually thicken the roux rather than dilute it, but don't worry, keep going) whisking all the while. You should have a thick sauce that easily coats the back of a spoon. Return to the heat and stir in the grated cheese. On a gentle heat, the cheese should melt and be incorporated into the sauce quite easily. If it isn't melting, turn the heat up a little. Finally, season with salt, pepper and grated nutmeg.

Arrange the chicken pieces in the bottom of a buttered, shallow ovenproof dish along with the florets of broccoli.

Put the Béchamel sauce, chicken stock and tarragon into a saucepan and reduce until you have about half the amount, then add the wine, cream and nutmeg. Finally, season to taste. You should have a creamy sauce on the thick side. Remove from the heat. Gradually add the Parmesan, a bit at a time, tasting all the while. You want a subtle flavour that's not overpowered by the cheese. Pour the sauce over the chicken and broccoli and scatter with ground almonds. Melt the butter and pour it over the dish.

Bake in the oven until you can see the gratin bubbling at the edges and the chicken has had a chance to heat through properly – about 15–20 minutes.

Nutritional value per serving

Calories 875 | Total Fat 62g | Sat Fat 16g | Carbs 33g | Fibre 2.5g | Protein 30g

Date	Time	Blood glucose level before meal	Blood glucose level 2 hours after meal	After-meal blood glucose on target (y/n)?	Notes, e.g. any changes made to recipe or portion size

THREE BEAN SALAD

You can serve this simple salad as a main dish or as the best possible accompaniment to Chilli Con Carne (page 169), substituting it for the typically served rice. It's also very versatile; swap the haricot beans for black-eyed beans for example. Use canned beans for ease, but if you prefer to use dried, you will need to soak them well in advance and cook them in plenty of boiling water and then allow to cool. Follow the instructions on the packets.

Serves 4

100g (4oz) canned chickpeas, rinsed and drained
100g (4oz) canned haricot beans, rinsed and drained
100g (4oz) canned red kidney beans, rinsed and drained
6–8 spring onions, chopped on the diagonal
½ medium red onion, finely sliced
1 tbsp good-quality red wine vinegar
250ml (9fl oz) extra-virgin olive oil
2 tbsp chopped parsley, to serve
2 tbsp chopped chives, to serve
salt and freshly ground black pepper, to taste

When you are ready to assemble the dish, simply mix all the ingredients in a bowl, season with salt and pepper and place in the fridge for an hour or two to chill. When ready to serve, finish with an extra sprinkling of parsley and chives.

Tip

Be careful with dried red kidney beans, as they will dye the water as they soak and cook, staining anything cooked with them.

Nutritional value per serving

Calories 380 | Total Fat 36g | Sat Fat 5g | Carbs 15g | Fibre 4g | Protein 5g

Date	Time	Blood glucose level before meal	Blood glucose level 2 hours after meal	After-meal blood glucose on target (y/n)?	Notes, e.g. any changes made to recipe or portion size

CHILLI CON CARNE

Originally made of dried beef mashed with dried chilli peppers, salt and suet and then made into small sun-dried bricks for reconstitution on the trail, chilli con carne is now the official dish of US State of Texas. There are a hundreds of recipes for this – with and without tomatoes. This particular one has stood the test of time. This is definitely one of those dishes that you can keep for a day or two in the fridge, reheating when needed. It somehow tastes even more scrumptious twenty-four hours after cooking.

Serves 4

2 tbsp extra-virgin rapeseed oil

600g (1lb 5oz) beef mince (or stewing steak chopped into small bite-sized pieces)

2 tbsp extra-virgin olive oil

1 large onion, roughly chopped

3 garlic cloves, crushed

1 tsp chilli powder

400g (14oz) can chopped tomatoes

2 tbsp tomato purée

600ml (1 pint) chicken stock

1 green pepper, deseeded and diced

400g (14oz) can red kidney beans

salt and freshly ground black pepper, to taste

In a large heavy-based pan heat the rapeseed oil to a high temperature and brown the meat in batches, stirring it regularly. Remove the meat from the pan and pour off any excess oil. Add the olive oil to the pan and on a gentle heat cook the onion until translucent. Now add the garlic, stir through and cook for a further 2–3 minutes, but don't allow the garlic to colour.

Return the meat to the pan, stir well and with the heat raised a little, cook for a few minutes. Add the chilli powder and stir it in. Add the tomatoes and cook for a further 5 minutes.

Meanwhile, add the tomato purée to the chicken stock, making sure it is well incorporated.

Pour sufficient stock into the meat until the sauce is wet, but not too watery. Put the lid on and over a low heat cook for 1 hour, stirring occasionally.

At the end of the hour, add the peppers, kidney beans and a good twist of black pepper. Cook, partially covered, for 30 minutes until you have an almost dry consistency. Remove from the heat, adjust the seasoning and serve with a freshly made salad.

Nutritional value per serving
Calories 600 | Total Fat 38g | Sat Fat 12g | Carbs 26g | Fibre 8g | Protein 41g

Main Meals

Date	Time	Blood glucose level before meal	Blood glucose level 2 hours after meal	After-meal blood glucose on target (y/n)?	Notes, e.g. any changes made to recipe or portion size

STIR-FRIED CHINESE LEAVES

Sometimes known as Peking cabbage, Chinese leaves have a wonderfully crunchy texture and seem to absorb the flavours of the ingredients they are cooked with.

Serves 2

2 tbsp peanut oil

1 large garlic clove, finely sliced

6 spring onions, finely cut on the diagonal

1 heaped tbsp freshly grated ginger

300g (10½oz) Chinese leaves, tough stalks removed,
*   leaves shredded*

1 tbsp dry sherry

1 tbsp soy sauce

2 tbsp chicken stock

salt

Heat the oil in a wok or large frying pan over a high heat until very hot. Add the garlic, onions and ginger. Stir-fry with a wooden spoon (or chopsticks) for 1 minute. This will flavour the oil. Throw in the Chinese leaves, sprinkle with 1 teaspoon of salt and keep moving and turning everything in the pan for 3 minutes. All the leaves should be coated in the oil.

Now add the sherry, soy sauce and 1 level tablespoon of the chicken stock. Lower the heat and cook for 2–3 minutes. If the leaves look like they are in a soup, raise the heat, if, on the other hand, they look like they are about to burn, add more stock by the spoonful. You should finish with a tiny but noticeable amount of juice and crisp tender cabbage.

Before serving, check and adjust the seasoning to taste.

Tip

All manner of leafy vegetables, singly or in combination, can be prepared in this way. Try spinach, leeks, Swiss chard, cabbages of any type, and even peas. You simply have to watch the timings to ensure they are cooked to perfection.

Nutritional value per serving

Calories 178 | Total Fat 14g | Sat Fat 3g | Carbs 8g | Fibre 2.7g | Protein 45g

Date	Time	Blood glucose level before meal	Blood glucose level 2 hours after meal	After-meal blood glucose on target (y/n)?	Notes (e.g. any changes made to recipe or portion size)

TUNA STEAKS WITH CUCUMBER AND TOMATO-FLAVOURED MAYONNAISE

Tuna and cucumber is a food marriage made in heaven, and in fact many such recorded recipes go back to the 1890s. This is a simple combination, so simple that it seems opportune to liven things up by adding a recipe for home-made mayonnaise, although you can, of course, use a shop-bought version.

Serves 4
55ml (2fl oz) extra-virgin olive oil
4 x 200g (7oz) tuna steaks
1 heaped tsp cayenne pepper
*¾ medium cucumber, peeled, seeds removed and flesh
    cut into 1cm (½in) rings,*
salt and freshly ground black pepper, to taste

For the mayonnaise:
2 large egg yolks at room temperature
generous pinch of salt
250ml (9fl oz) extra-virgin olive oil
1 tsp white wine vinegar or lemon juice
1 tsp Dijon mustard
1 large tomato, skinned and deseeded
1 tbsp unsalted butter

Put the olive oil in a food bag, add the steaks and the cayenne and black peppers. Rub the steaks with the spices and oil to ensure they are well covered. Set aside for 30 minutes.

Poach the cucumber rings in a pan of lightly boiling salted water for 15 minutes until tender. Refresh in a colander under cold running water and tip onto a clean tea towel to drain.

Heat a griddle pan or heavy-based frying pan on a high heat and once really hot, cook each steak for 2 minutes, turn it over then cook the other side for 2 minutes. Repeat. A 'meaty' fish like tuna is best served slightly 'pink' rather than entirely cooked through, but it's a matter of choice. Place the steaks on a warm plate, cover with tin foil and let them stand for 5 minutes.

Next make the mayonnaise. Put the egg yolks in a large mixing bowl and beat well with a whisk for 2–3 minutes before adding the salt and continuing to beat for another 30 seconds until the yolks have thickened. Pour the oil into the bowl in a very (very) thin stream, or drop by drop if you don't have a second pair of hands to help, beating all of the time. Do not, under any circumstance, rush this process; if you do, your mayonnaise will split. As you approach the consistency you want (you may not need all of the oil), continue to beat for another 30 seconds until you have something in the bowl that is thick and glossy. Add the white wine vinegar (or lemon juice) and mustard and gently mix in. If you need to thin the mixture a little, add a few drops of cold water.

Cook the tomato in butter for a few minutes and season well with salt and pepper. Allow to cool, chop and stir into the mayonnaise.

Place each steak on top of a portion of the cucumber rings and dot the mayonnaise around them liberally.

Tip
Make sure that all the mayonnaise ingredients are at room temperature before you start.

Nutritional value per serving
Calories 644 | Total Fat 56g | Sat Fat 9g | Carbs 5g | Fibre 1g | Protein 58g

Date	Time	Blood glucose level before meal	Blood glucose level 2 hours after meal	After-meal blood glucose on target (y/n)?	Notes (e.g. any changes made to recipe or portion size)

SPANISH TORTILLA

A Spanish tortilla is a close culinary cousin to the Persian kuku. Both are omelette-like egg-based dishes containing two or more vegetables that are cooked on the hob and finished under the grill to give an almost solid quality. It can be eaten hot or cold and makes great picnic food. People in Spain argue endlessly whether to add onion or not. You can decide for yourself, but well-caramelised onions certainly add to the flavour. A pinch of cayenne pepper will liven up the dish no end.

Serves 4
8 eggs
*2 medium potatoes, peeled and cut into 1cm (½in)
    chunks (optional)*
splash of Worcestershire sauce (optional)
3 tbsp extra-virgin olive oil
1 large Spanish onion, sliced
*other fillings or your choice, such as spinach, green
    pepper; broccoli florets, peas (frozen or fresh), pieces
    of ham or chorizo sausage*
½–1 tsp cayenne pepper (optional)
salt and freshly ground black pepper, to taste

Preheat the grill to high. Beat the eggs in a large bowl and season well with salt and pepper.

If you are going to include potatoes, parboil them in a pan of boiling salted water for 10 minutes or until a knife easily penetrates. Drain and allow them to sit gently steaming; they will soon dry out, which is what you want. Then sauté them in olive oil for 5 or so minutes, finishing them off with a splash of Worcestershire sauce, if you like. Any other vegetables you plan to include should be cooked until *al dente* rather than mushy.

Add the olive oil to a heavy-based pan and when hot add the onion slices. Cook for 5–7 minutes, stirring occasionally, until they brown. Add the potato, cooked vegetables and any other fillings and stir through. Cook for 3 minutes. Using a slotted spoon, so that the oil drips back into the pan, transfer the contents of the pan into the bowl of whisked eggs and stir through so everything is well mixed.

Reheat the oil in the pan and once hot pour in the egg and vegetable mixture. Smooth it out with the back of a wooden spoon until you have an even, thick cake (add the cayenne pepper at this stage, if you like). Cook on a medium heat for 5–7 minutes or until it appears well set and then place under a hot grill for another 5 minutes until it is nicely browned and there is no liquid egg on top.

Serve hot, warm or cold. It goes particularly well with a plate of sautéed kidneys.

Tip

To lower the carb content, you can dispense with the potato and substitute it with a firm vegetable like broccoli. You won't have an authentic tortilla, but you will still have a chunky tasty slice of Spanish goodness.

Nutritional value per serving

Calories 320 | Total Fat 21g | Sat Fat 5g | Carbs 21g | Fibre 2.6g | Protein 15g

Date	Time	Blood glucose level before meal	Blood glucose level 2 hours after meal	After-meal blood glucose on target (y/n)?	Notes (e.g. any changes made to recipe or portion size)

TOMATO SALAD

A salad should be hymn to the quality of its ingredients. Take tomatoes – there is a world of difference between the soggy, flavourless example often found in supermarkets and one from a home-grown, sun-blessed and juicily ripe crop. Or you can search out heritage varieties (sometimes called 'heirloom') at farmers' markets.

Serves 4

12 or so good-quality, ripe, medium-sized tomatoes, sliced
1 medium red onion, cut in half and thinly sliced
a few basil leaves, torn
salt and freshly ground black pepper, to taste

For the vinaigrette
50ml (1¾fl oz) white or red wine vinegar
1 tsp Dijon or grain mustard
250ml (9fl oz) extra-virgin olive oil

To make the vinaigrette pour the vinegar into a small bowl. Add the mustard along with a pinch of salt and plenty of pepper, stir, then pour in the extra-virgin olive oil.

Place the tomatoes neatly on a serving plate then sprinkle with a good dose of coarsely ground black pepper. Scatter the onion over the tomatoes and douse with the vinaigrette.

Finally, top with a handful of freshly torn basil leaves. The perfect autumn salad.

Tip

If you prefer you can use a good-quality balsamic vinegar in place of the white or red wine vinegar, in which case go easy on the salt and pepper and leave out the mustard; balsamic vinegar has more than enough flavour on its own.

Some variants:
With egg

Top a layer of sliced tomatoes seasoned with black pepper with a layer of sliced hard-boiled eggs likewise seasoned. Repeat with another layer of tomatoes and eggs.

Sprinkle with chopped parsley and chives to finish, and a liberal splash of white wine vinegar vinaigrette.

With tuna

Make a tomato and egg salad as above and season it with white wine vinegar vinaigrette.

In a bowl, mix a can of tuna with a couple of tablespoons of mayonnaise and some chopped chives (and a chopped spring onion, if you like). Season with salt and pepper to taste.

Nutritional value per serving of tomato salad

Calories 488 | Total Fat 48g | Sat Fat 7g | Carbs 19g | Fibre 4.5g | Protein 3.5g

Reverse Your Diabetes Diet

Date	Time	Blood glucose level before meal	Blood glucose level 2 hours after meal	After-meal blood glucose on target (y/n)?	Notes (e.g. any changes made to recipe or portion size)

NAVARIN OF LAMB
(NAVARIN PRINTANIER)

This wonderful stew of lamb with young spring vegetables is thought to be so-called in honour of the Battle of Navarino in 1827, which ended the Greek War of Independence and was the last naval battle fought by sailing ships. Prosaically, the name is more likely to refer to the traditional inclusion of turnips (*navet*, in French) in the dish. Either way, good-quality lamb and fresh vegetables make this spring stew a delight. Traditionally, this recipe would contain new potatoes. Of course you can cook them separately and serve them to those who wish to indulge, otherwise just enjoy the carrots and turnips which have a much lower carb content.

Serves 4

1kg (2¼lb) boned shoulder of lamb or neck fillet,
    cut into chunks
3 tbsp extra-virgin olive oil
1 large onion, quartered
70g (2½oz) tomato purée
400g (14oz) can plum tomatoes, chopped
1 large garlic clove, roughly chopped
500ml (17½fl oz) vegetable stock
pinch of cayenne
sprig of rosemary (or 1 tsp dried)
sprig of thyme (or 1 tsp dried)
1 bay leaf

10–12 small carrots, topped, tailed and scrubbed
6 baby turnips, scrubbed and cut in half
bunch of parsley, chopped, to serve
salt and freshly ground black pepper, to taste

Season the lamb well with salt and pepper. Heat a heavy-based pan, add the diced meat and brown all over with the lid on. You may have to do this in batches. Set the lamb aside in a warm place. Pour off the fat that will have accumulated in the pan and dispose of it when it has cooled sufficiently.

In the same pan, heat the olive oil and cook the onion until soft, then add the tomato purée, tomatoes, garlic and stock. Add a good amount of black pepper, a pinch of cayenne pepper, the rosemary, thyme and bay leaf. Cover and bring to the boil, turn the heat down and simmer for 15 minutes. Add the carrots and turnips, cover, and simmer for a 10 minutes.

Return the meat to the pan, bring everything back to the boil and then simmer with the lid on for about 1 hour or until the meat is tender and the vegetables are well cooked. If the dish looks a little too watery, leave the lid off for the last 10 minutes or so, but be careful not to dry it out too much. Serve immediately with plenty of chopped parsley sprinkled over the top.

Nutritional value per serving
Calories 746 | Total Fat 52g | Sat Fat 23g | Carbs 22g | Fibre 6g | Protein 48g

Main Meals

Date	Time	Blood glucose level before meal	Blood glucose level 2 hours after meal	After-meal blood glucose on target (y/n)?	Notes (e.g. any changes made to recipe or portion size)

KOZHI KURUMULAGU (SPICY SOUTHERN INDIAN BLACK PEPPER CHICKEN)

This is perhaps the most famous dish of the Travancore region of the state of Kerala, in southern India. Kerala has been a worldwide exporter of spices since 3000 BCE, and this peppery dish is a testament to the rich-tasting food of southern Indian cooking – somewhat different in character to the usual Bengali fare found in so many restaurants in Britain, because the heat in the dish comes from the black pepper rather than chilli.

This recipe was supplied by the chef of the Kayal restaurant group based in the West Midlands, which specialises in healthy south Indian food (www. kayalrestaurant.com).

Serves 4

3 green cardamom pods, very lightly crushed

1 tsp fennel seeds

2 cinnamon sticks

3 cloves

2 heaped tbsp black peppercorns

1 tsp melted ghee

2 heaped tbsp cashew nut kernels

2 tbsp ghee or clarified butter (see page 124)

1 tsp mustard seeds

6 shallots or 2 medium-sized Indian onions, finely chopped

2½cm (1in) piece of fresh root ginger, finely chopped
4 garlic cloves, finely chopped
small handful of curry leaves, finely chopped, plus extra
   to garnish
3 tsp ground coriander
2 level tsp turmeric
5 medium tomatoes, skinned and finely chopped
1kg (2¼lb) boneless chicken meat, cut into small bite-
   sized chunks
250ml (8¾fl oz) coconut milk
salt, to taste

Begin by toasting the cardamom, fennel, cinnamon and cloves in a small heavy-based frying pan until the spices begin to brown and release their aromatic oils. Remove the pan from the heat and allow the spices to cool before grinding them to a powder in a spice or coffee grinder (or a pestle and mortar, but you will need plenty of elbow grease).

To make the black pepper paste, put the black peppercorns in a spice (or coffee) grinder and blitz briefly until you have a coarse gritty powder. Add 1 tablespoon of water and stir before adding the melted ghee, then stir again and set aside.

To make the cashew paste, boil the cashew nut kernels in a small saucepan for 5 minutes. Drain and blitz very briefly in a small food processor. Add 1 tablespoon of water and blitz again; you should end up with a very smooth paste.

Heat the ghee or butter in a deep heavy-based pan until hot then add the mustard seeds. They will start to ping about, and once they do, lower the heat and add the shallots (or onions). Cook for 4–5 minutes until translucent and then add the ginger, garlic and curry leaves. Give everything a good stir and cook for 2 minutes. Then add the coriander, turmeric and 4 tablespoons of the black pepper paste and cook for 3 minutes. Add in the tomatoes and cook on a medium heat until the sauce in the pan begins to thicken. Add the roasted and ground spice mixture to the pan, stir everything and cook for 5 minutes with the lid off.

Now add the chicken to the pan with a little salt and cook, stirring, until the chicken has turned white and is on its way to being cooked. Add enough water to cover the chicken, put a lid on and cook for 15 minutes or until the chicken is nearly cooked. Add 4 tablespoons of the cashew paste and the coconut milk and keep on the heat until the chicken is fully cooked. You should end up with quite a wet (almost broth-like) sauce. Check the seasoning, garnish with a few curry leaves and serve immediately.

Nutritional value per serving
Calories 586 | Total Fat 32g | Sat Fat 7g | Carbs 18g | Fibre 2g | Protein 65g

Main Meals

Date	Time	Blood glucose level before meal	Blood glucose level 2 hours after meal	After-meal blood glucose on target (y/n)?	Notes (e.g. any changes made to recipe or portion size)

'COUSCOUS MADE
MY NEIGHBOUR'S WAY'

A recipe by Jean-Christophe Novelli

Jean-Christophe Novelli is a multi-Michelin-starred chef who focuses on using quality produce and natural ingredients. This is a dish that he has created especially for this book to honour his father (who has diabetes). It is delicious and could grace any fine dining table.

Serves 6

1 tbsp extra-virgin olive oil
1kg (2¼lbs) neck of lamb fillet, cut into large dice
2 chicken legs, cut through the joint to create 4 pieces
2 medium onions, peeled and quartered
4 baby carrots, scrubbed and trimmed
2 baby turnips, halved lengthways
300g (10½oz) celeriac, peeled and cut into large dice
50g (1¾oz) fresh ginger, peeled and thinly sliced
1 tsp coriander seeds
½ tsp turmeric
1 tsp cumin seeds
½ bulb garlic
400g (14oz) can chopped tomatoes
200g (7oz) can flageolet beans (or 200g (7oz) fresh broad beans when in season)
2 tbsp tomato purée
500ml (17½fl oz) hot lamb or vegetable stock

1 courgette, chopped into large pieces
1 aubergine, chopped into large pieces
1 bulb fennel, quartered and diced
1 tbsp harissa paste
a few fresh green herbs to garnish, such as parsley
    and a little chopped thyme
salt and freshly ground black pepper

For the couscous:
300g (10½oz) couscous, cooked
3 tbsp extra-virgin olive oil
½ tsp mild curry powder
½ tsp turmeric
300ml (10fl oz) hot lamb or vegetable stock

Heat a little extra-virgin olive oil in a deep pan and seal the lamb, then add the chicken pieces and seal. Tip in the onions, carrots, turnips, celeriac and ginger. Place the lid on the pan and shake the ingredients to combine. Next, add the coriander seeds, turmeric, cumin seeds, the garlic and the tomatoes. Stir, then add the flageolet (or broad) beans and the tomato purée and stir again. Add the stock to cover everything in the pan, cover with the lid and bring to the boil. Reduce the heat and simmer.

After 30 minutes of cooking, add the rest of the vegetables and bring back to a simmer (don't allow it to boil at all). Cover and leave to simmer for 30 minutes. Taste the sauce and adjust the seasoning. At this point, add the harissa and continue to simmer for a further 30 minutes.

Meanwhile, prepare the couscous. Using a stainless-steel or large glass bowl, mix the couscous and the olive oil with your hands. Add the curry powder and turmeric, then pour in the stock. Stir with a fork and cover with cling film. After 10 minutes or so, the couscous can be stirred lightly with the fork to break up any clumps.

When the stew is ready, place the couscous on a large serving plate or bowl. Spoon the meat and vegetables into the middle of the dish and decorate with green herbs. Serve immediately.

Nutritional value per serving

Calories 724 | Total Fat 46g | Sat Fat 17g | Carbs 40g | Fibre 7.2g | Protein 43g

Date	Time	Blood glucose level before meal	Blood glucose level 2 hours after meal	After-meal blood glucose on target (y/n)?	Notes (e.g. any changes made to recipe or portion size)

MONKFISH WITH SAFFRON SAUCE

It has to be said that the monkfish would be a distant last in any beauty competition, but the edible part (the tail) has a succulent meaty flesh that is absolutely delicious. If you are having a special occasion, this Italian-style recipe is just the ticket. Perfect with crunchy steamed green beans.

Serves 4

800g (1¾lbs) monkfish, cleaned, skin, membrane and bones removed and cut into 4 pieces

1 x court bouillon (see page 211)

30g (1oz) unsalted butter, plus a further 30g (1oz), well chilled and diced

1 shallot (or small onion), finely chopped

400ml (14fl oz) hot fish stock

1 glass white wine

grated nutmeg

pinch of saffron

bunch of flat-leaf parsley, chopped

salt and freshly ground black pepper

See how to make a court bouillon on page 211. Place the fish in a deep pan, cover with the bouillon and very gently bring to the boil. Immediately turn the heat right down so just a few bubbles are rising to the surface. Put on a tight-fitting lid and poach the fish for 15–20 minutes.

Meanwhile, make the sauce. Heat the first 30g (1oz) of the butter in a pan and gently cook the shallot (or onion) until it is softened and translucent. Add the hot fish stock and wine and reduce over a high heat until you have about half the volume of liquid. Remove from the heat and pour through a sieve. Return the sauce to the pan and add a small amount of grated nutmeg and the saffron.

While still on the heat, slowly add the small cubes of chilled butter, beating briskly. The butter should emulsify and thicken the sauce. Keep adding the butter, one cube at a time until it is all incorporated and you have a smooth, shiny sauce. Adjust the seasoning and set aside in a warm place. It can be gently reheated when it's time to serve.

When everything is ready, gently spoon 2–3 tablespoons of sauce onto warmed plates, place a piece of the fish on top and sprinkle with the chopped parsley.

Nutritional value per serving
Calories 283 | Total Fat 12g | Sat Fat 5g | Carbs 6g | Fibre 1g | Protein 31g

Date	Time	Blood glucose level before meal	Blood glucose level 2 hours after meal	After-meal blood glucose on target (y/n)?	Notes (e.g. any changes made to recipe or portion size)

SICILIAN-STYLE TUNA

Tuna steaks are a treat. The meat is moderately high in fat and has a firmly textured flaky but tender flesh, making it ideal for grilling, frying or stewing as in this recipe.

Serves 4
100ml (3½fl oz) extra-virgin olive oil
4 x 200g (7oz) tuna steaks (as fresh as possible)
1 red pepper, deseeded and cut into 1cm (½in) strips
2 garlic cloves, finely chopped
4 large tomatoes, skinned, deseeded and chopped
2 tbsp black olives
1 tsp dried oregano (or a handful of fresh leaves, chopped)
sprig of rosemary
1 dried red chilli, crushed
1 bay leaf
1 small glass of Marsala (for authenticity)
    or use 1 large glass of a not-too-dry white wine
salt and freshly ground black pepper

Begin by heating some of the olive oil in a heavy-based pan and briefly fry the tuna steaks on both sides to seal in the juices. Remove the steaks with a slotted spoon or tongs and set aside in a warm place covered with tin foil.

Return the pan to the heat, replenish the olive oil if necessary, and fry the pepper strips for 5–7 minutes until they start to soften. Add the garlic and cook for 3 minutes, but do not let the garlic colour. Add the tomatoes, olives, oregano, rosemary, crushed chilli and bay leaf. Stir in the Marsala or white wine and return the tuna to the pan. Make sure the sauce covers the steaks. Cover the pan with the lid and allow it to gently simmer for 15–20 minutes. At the end, the tuna should be tender and the sauce fresh tasting. Adjust the seasoning, being generous with the pepper, and serve immediately. *Buon appetito!*

Nutritional value per serving
Calories 490 | Total Fat 26.5g | Sat Fat 4g | Carbs 11g | Fibre 2.6g | Protein 49g

Date	Time	Blood glucose level before meal	Blood glucose level 2 hours after meal	After-meal blood glucose on target (y/n)?	Notes (e.g. any changes made to recipe or portion size)

CALF'S LIVER WITH SAGE

Simplicity itself, but a sublime combination that has stood, and will continue to stand, the test of culinary time. Serve with plenty of runner beans or broad beans and perhaps a dash of Worcestershire sauce.

Serves 4
600g (1lb 5oz) calf's liver, cut into 4 pieces
50g (1¾oz) flour, for dusting
50g (1¾oz) unsalted butter
12 fresh sage leaves
salt and freshly ground black pepper, to taste

Season the liver with salt and pepper and then coat lightly in the flour.

Heat the butter to the point that it is foaming (but don't let it brown) in a heavy-based pan. Fry the liver pieces for 2–3 minutes on one side, then turn over and add the sage leaves. Cook for another 2–3 minutes and serve immediately on warm plates.

Nutritional value per serving
Calories 377 | Total Fat 21g | Sat Fat 6g | Carbs 13g | Fibre 1.5g | Protein 33g

Reverse Your Diabetes Diet

Date	Time	Blood glucose level before meal	Blood glucose level 2 hours after meal	After-meal blood glucose on target (y/n)?	Notes (e.g. any changes made to recipe or portion size)

LA PARMIGIANA DI MELANZANE (AUBERGINE PARMESAN)

This is a dish you will find served all over northern Italy and is both rustic and robust. Its bold flavours will fill you with warmth and good cheer and is the perfect dish to share with family and friends. Just stick to a modest portion size and resist the yearnings for seconds.

As with all century-old recipes there is plenty of debate about the method, and you can find variants that dispense with either pressing the aubergine or frying it in oil, but this method is about as traditional as it gets.

Serves 4

2 large eggs

4 small aubergines, sliced into ¾cm (⅓in) roundels and salted (see page 161)

30g (1oz) plain flour, for dusting

4 tbsp olive oil

2 x 125g (4½oz) packs mozzarella cheese, chopped into bite-sized pieces

150g (5oz) grated Parmesan

salt and freshly ground black pepper, to taste

For the tomato sauce:

55ml (2fl oz) extra-virgin olive oil

2 garlic cloves, finely chopped

400g (14oz) can plum tomatoes

400g (14oz) can chopped tomatoes or 650g (1½lbs)
   tomatoes, skinned, deseeded and chopped
1 glass red wine (optional)
8–10 fresh basil leaves, torn (or 1 heaped tsp of dried
   basil)

Preheat the oven to 180°C/350°F/gas mark 4.

First make the tomato sauce. Put the olive oil in a deep heavy-based saucepan and heat gently. Add the garlic and cook for 3 minutes, stirring all the time. Once it starts to take on a golden colour remove the pan from the heat and add all the tomatoes. Return to the heat and bring to a gentle bubble, breaking up the plum tomatoes and stirring all the time. Add the wine, if using, partially cover and cook on a medium heat for 30 minutes. Finally, add the basil and season carefully – Parmesan will add a pronounced salty note to the dish.

Break the eggs into a jug, add salt and pepper and lightly whisk. Lightly dust a batch of aubergines in flour and dip into the egg. Fry the aubergines in a heavy-based frying pan in the olive oil until they are golden brown on both sides. Pile them up on kitchen paper to drain and keep going until all the aubergines are prepared. There is no way around the facts that (a) the aubergines will soak up an extraordinary amount of oil and (b) this is a time- and labour-intensive process that can't be rushed.

To assemble the dish, spoon a layer of the tomato sauce on the bottom of an ovenproof dish (a lasagne dish is ideal), top with a layer of aubergine and dot with mozzarella. Spoon tomato sauce over the mozzarella and then sprinkle over about a quarter of the Parmesan. Continue with another layer of aubergine, mozzarella, tomato sauce and Parmesan. Hopefully you will have judged the quantities so that you can construct three layers of aubergine, mozzarella and sauce, finishing with an especially generous covering of Parmesan. Bake in the oven for 30–40 minutes then allow to stand for 10 minutes before serving. (This is even better after it has been in the fridge overnight, served cold the next day.)

Nutritional value per serving
Calories 482 | Total Fat 32g | Sat Fat 21g | Carbs 18g | Fibre 4.4g | Protein 44g

Date	Time	Blood glucose level before meal	Blood glucose level 2 hours after meal	After-meal blood glucose on target (y/n)?	Notes (e.g. any changes made to recipe or portion size)

GRILLED MACKEREL WITH WHITE WINE VINEGAR

The mackerel is a fish we should all eat a great deal more of. Identifiable by its iridescent silver-and-blue-striped skin it is firm of flesh, oil-rich and intensely flavoured. Highly nutritious, it is easy to prepare and is endlessly versatile: it can be grilled, fried or barbecued, and when stuffed with aromatic herbs it is perfect for baking in the oven. It also is fabulous in curry dishes.

Freshness is everything with fish – only buy what's on the slab if the fish's skin remains iridescent, has firm flesh when poked and looks at you with bright, shiny engaging eyes.

Serves 4

4 x 220g (7¾oz) fresh mackerel
55g (2oz) unsalted butter
200ml (7fl oz) good-quality cider, white wine
    or sherry vinegar
salad and wholemeal toast, to serve (optional)
salt and freshly ground black pepper, to taste

Preheat the grill and season the flesh of the mackerel well with salt and pepper.

Heat the butter in a heavy-based pan on a medium heat until it is frothing but has not turned brown. Place each fillet in the pan (you will need to pack them in or do it in batches) skin side down and, pressing with a fish slice, cook for about 4 minutes.

Now pour in the vinegar, spoon the melted butter over the fillets and place under the grill and cook for a couple of minutes until cooked through.

Remove the fillets to serving plates and pour the juices from the pan over each fillet. Serve with salad and some wholemeal toast, if you like.

Tip

If you can get your fishmonger to fillet the mackerel, it will save you a job, but it's not too difficult to do at home if you have a sharp knife with a point.

Make a diagonal cut parallel to the line of the gills behind the pectoral fin of the fish until you feel the knife touch the backbone. Then turn it over and repeat on the other side. Put the fish belly side down and cut through the backbone removing the head. With the fish placed side down on the cutting board, run the knife down one side of the backbone, keeping as close to it as you can. With a sawing motion cut the fillet away, always keeping as close to the backbone as possible. Set the fillet aside. Now flip over the fish and repeat on the other side of the backbone. Remove the pin-bones from the middle of the fillets with tweezers (spending time on this will much improve the experience of eating your fillets later on) and trim the fillet of any excess skin. Wash gently under cold running water, pat dry with kitchen paper and you are ready to go.

Nutritional value per serving
Calories 625 | Total Fat 48g | Sat Fat 14g | Carbs 0g |
Fibre 0g | Protein 46g

Date	Time	Blood glucose level before meal	Blood glucose level 2 hours after meal	After-meal blood glucose on target (y/n)?	Notes (e.g. any changes made to recipe or portion size)

MACKEREL WITH CORIANDER AND CHILLI, SERVED WITH A RED ONION AND TOMATO SALAD

Serves 4

2 garlic cloves, grated

3 tsp coriander seeds, crushed in a pestle and mortar

½ tsp chilli powder

1 tsp turmeric

1 tsp black peppercorn, crushed in a pestle and mortar

1 level tsp sea salt

125ml (4½fl oz) extra-virgin olive oil

4 x 220g (7¾oz) whole mackerel, gutted

For the salad

10 small tomatoes, cut in halves or quarters

1 medium red onion, finely sliced

2 tbsp chopped coriander leaves

225g (8oz) black-eyed beans, rinsed and drained

50ml (1¾fl oz) extra-virgin olive oil

juice of ½ lime

First prepare the marinade. Combine the garlic, coriander, chilli, turmeric, crushed peppercorns and sea salt in a bowl. Pour in the olive oil and stir everything together.

Place each fish on a cutting board and make 3 or 4 small diagonal incisions in the flesh. Turn over and repeat. Put the whole fish into the bowl with the marinade and massage with your fingers so that the marinade is rubbed well into the incisions. Cover the bowl with cling film and place in the fridge for at least 30 minutes.

While the fish is marinating, make the salad. Put all the chopped ingredients in a bowl along with the black-eyed beans, olive oil and lime juice. Mix well together and chill in the fridge while you cook the fish.

Heat a griddle pan or heavy-based frying pan on a high heat until the pan is hot. Add the fish and cook for 5 or 6 minutes on each side. The skin should be well charred and the flesh nicely cooked without it drying out. Serve immediately with the chilled salad.

Nutritional value per serving
Calories 1008 | Total Fat 82g | Sat Fat 14g | Carbs 25g | Fibre 7.7g | Protein 54g

Date	Time	Blood glucose level before meal	Blood glucose level 2 hours after meal	After-meal blood glucose on target (y/n)?	Notes (e.g. any changes made to recipe or portion size)

PAN-FRIED MACKEREL SERVED WITH CUCUMBER AND CHILLI TAGLIATELLE

Serves 4

*1 medium cucumber, peeled, deseeded and flesh cut into
    ribbons with a peeler*
1 green chilli, deseeded and cut into small dice
8 spring onions, sliced diagonally
150ml (5¼fl oz) extra-virgin olive oil
4 x 220g (7¾oz) mackerel, filleted
juice of 1 lime
sea salt, to taste
small bunch of coriander, roughly chopped
brown bread, to serve

Put the cucumber 'tagliatelle' in a bowl and add half of
the chilli along with three-quarters of the spring onions.
Pour in 100ml (3½fl oz) or so of the olive oil and half the
lime juice and toss to mix well. Keep in the fridge until
you are ready to serve.

Add the remaining olive oil to a heavy-based frying
pan and heat so that the pan is really hot, but the oil is
not smoking. Season the flesh of the fillets with sea salt
and pack in as many fillets as will comfortably fit in the
pan, skin side down. Cook for 2–3 minutes until the skin
is crisp. Pour the remaining lime juice over the fillets and
turn them over in the pan. Cook for another 2 minutes
and lift the 8 fillets onto 4 warm plates. Sprinkle with the
remaining spring onions, chopped coriander and chilli

and serve with the cucumber salad and some brown bread to soak up the juices.

Nutritional value per serving

Calories 812 | Total Fat 68g | Sat Fat 12g | Carbs 6g | Fibre 2g | Protein 47g

Date	Time	Blood glucose level before meal	Blood glucose level 2 hours after meal	After-meal blood glucose on target (y/n)?	Notes (e.g. any changes made to recipe or portion size)

THE PERFECT ROAST COD

There remain real concerns about eating cod as over-fishing in the 80s and 90s reduced some stocks in the North Atlantic to dangerously low levels. With the introduction of rigorously enforced quotas, the good news is that there is scientific evidence that stocks are recovering. That said, always buy line-caught fish from sustainable fisheries that carry the Marine Stewardship Council's (MSC) blue tick logo. Or you can use haddock here and prepare it in just the same way.

Serves 4

75g (2½oz) unsalted butter
3 tbsp extra-virgin olive oil
4 x 200g (7oz) thick cod fillets, the thicker the better
salt and freshly ground black pepper, to taste

Preheat the oven to 200°C/400°F/gas mark 6.

In a deep heavy-based ovenproof frying pan (suitable for use in the oven) heat the olive oil and the butter, letting it melt, froth and bubble. Season the fish fillets with plenty of salt and pepper and place in the hot butter and oil, skin side down. Using a fish slice to keep flat, cook for about 2 minutes until the skin is nice and brown. Turn the fillets over, put the pan in the oven and bake for 8–10 minutes until the flesh in the middle of each fillet is entirely opaque.

Serve on warmed plates with the juices from the pan and plenty of buttered spinach.

Nutritional value per serving
Calories 421 | Total Fat 28g | Sat Fat 11g | Carbs 4g | Fibre 0g | Protein 34g

Date	Time	Blood glucose level before meal	Blood glucose level 2 hours after meal	After-meal blood glucose on target (y/n)?	Notes (e.g. any changes made to recipe or portion size)

POACHED SALMON

A poached salmon quietly residing in your fridge, just waiting to be cut into wedges is always worth the investment in time and money. It makes a quick and easy lunch when eaten with a green salad or with mayonnaise, watercress and brown bread and butter.

There are two schools of thought about the poaching method: in salted water or in a court bouillon. Repeated blind tests demonstrate that no one can tell the difference, so adopt whichever process feels right.

Serves plenty
1 whole salmon, gutted, descaled and washed

For the court bouillon
1 onion, peeled and quartered
1 carrot, peeled and roughly chopped
1 celery stick, washed, trimmed and roughly chopped
3 sprigs of thyme
small bunch of parsley
1 bay leaf
1 tsp black peppercorns
1 tsp coriander seeds
3 tbsp salt
3 litres (5 pints) cold water

To make the court bouillon, add all the ingredients to the water in a large saucepan. Bring to the boil, lower the heat and simmer, uncovered, for 40 minutes. Strain through a sieve and there you have it. The court bouillon can be kept in the refrigerator for up to 3 days or will freeze for several months. Always use it cold.

If you are using salt water to cook your fish the ratio should be in the order of 50g (1¾oz) salt per 1 litre (1¾ pints) of water.

To poach your salmon, make sure it is thoroughly descaled. Ideally the fishmonger will have done this for you, but it's worth running the back of a knife from the tail towards the head and tidying up the job. Wash the fish inside and out under cold running water before putting it into a large deep pan or an 'I use it once every two years' fish kettle. Tip in enough *cold* water or *cold* court bouillon to cover the fish, and very gently bring to the boil on the hob. Do not let it go past the few gentle bubbles stage before slapping on a tight-fitting lid and turning off the heat. Set it aside somewhere cool and out of the way and leave to continue cooking – preferably overnight. You will end up with a beautifully moist fish.

Carefully take the fish from the water/bouillon (which should be discarded as it is too salty to use for anything else), remove the skin of the fish (another one of those messy but satisfying jobs) and you are done.

Nutritional value per 200g (7oz) serving
Calories 321 | Total Fat 9g | Sat Fat 1.5g | Carbs 5g | Fibre 1.3g | Protein 52g

Main Meals

Date	Time	Blood glucose level before meal	Blood glucose level 2 hours after meal	After-meal blood glucose on target (y/n)?	Notes (e.g. any changes made to recipe or portion size)

PAN-FRIED DOVER SOLE

The Dover sole is an exquisite, meaty-textured flat fish, superior, by virtue of being more firm and flavoursome, than its cousins the lemon sole or the plaice – both of which can be cooked in the same manner. The Dover sole is a dinner-table extravagance and benefits from the simplest preparation – fried and coated in browned butter with a squeeze of lemon and served with a simple green salad or wilted greens.

Serves 2
2 x 450g (1lb) Dover sole, lemon sole or plaice, skin removed (see tip)
30g (1oz) plain flour, for dusting
2 tbsp extra-virgin olive oil
75g (2½oz) unsalted butter
1 lemon, juice of ½, ½ cut into wedges to serve
1 heaped tsp finely chopped parsley
sea salt and freshly ground black pepper, to taste

You know the famous film quote, *'We're gonna need a bigger boat'*? Well, to pan-fry a sole you're gonna need a bigger frying pan. Assuming you have one to hand, lightly dust the white-skinned side of the fish in flour and then brush with some of the olive oil. Season well with salt and pepper.

Heat the remaining olive oil in the pan on a medium heat and then place the fish white-skin side down and fry for 5–6 minutes. Carefully turn the fish over and fry for another 5 minutes. Remove from the pan and keep warm under foil.

Put the butter into the same pan, turn up the heat slightly and melt and cook until it turns a nutty brown colour (beyond the frothing stage). Season with salt and pepper, a good squeeze of lemon juice and add in the chopped parsley.

Place the fish on warmed serving plates, pour over the nut-brown butter and serve with a wedge of lemon.

Tip
To prepare the fish you will need to remove the dark skin. Make a cut near the tail with a very sharp knife and lift enough of the skin so you can get a good grip. Pull towards the head and the skin should come away cleanly. The white skin can be left on as it will crisp up nicely in the pan.

Nutritional value per serving
Calories 846 | Total Fat 50g | Sat Fat 22g | Carbs 13g | Fibre 1.2g | Protein 83g

Date	Time	Blood glucose level before meal	Blood glucose level 2 hours after meal	After-meal blood glucose on target (y/n)?	Notes (e.g. any changes made to recipe or portion size)

HALIBUT *EN PAPILLOTE*

En papillote is a great way of cooking fish. It literally means 'in parchment' or, as it is more usually translated, 'in a parcel'. Fish cooked this way, wrapped in a sort of paper bag, retain their moisture, flavour and all-important natural juices. Before you pop it into the oven, you can, of course, top the fish with all manner of herbs, lemons or specially created whatnots.

This method works just as well with plaice and pollock.

Serves 2

1 lemon, juice of ½, other ½ cut into fine slices
4 x 150g (5½oz) skinless and boneless halibut fillets cut
    from the thick end of the fish
2 tbsp extra-virgin olive oil
sea salt flakes and 1 tsp crushed white peppercorns
2 bay leaves
steamed cavolo nero, kale or spinach, to serve

Preheat the oven to 200°C/400°F/gas mark 6. Cut 2 pieces of greaseproof paper large enough (be generous) to fold under and over the fish to make a neat parcel with room at the top. The fish has to 'breathe' in the parcel.

Lay a couple of slices of lemon in the centre of each piece of greaseproof paper, place the fish on top, smear them with a good glug of olive oil and season with sea salt and crushed white peppercorns and pop the bay leaves on top. Fold over the paper until you have a tightly scrunched parcel, place on a baking tray and bake for 15 minutes until the fish is just cooked through.

Remove the fish from its paper parcel, being careful not to spill all the lovely oil and juices, which you should pour straight back over the fish. Give each one another good squeeze of lemon juice and serve with either steamed cavolo nero, kale or spinach.

Nutritional value per serving
Calories 440 | Total Fat 21g | Sat Fat 3.2g | Carbs 2g | Fibre 0g | Protein 60g

Date	Time	Blood glucose level before meal	Blood glucose level 2 hours after meal	After-meal blood glucose on target (y/n)?	Notes (e.g. any changes made to recipe or portion size)

DESSERTS

I have deliberately not included any recipes for desserts as by definition most contain sugar, something I would encourage you to avoid as much as possible. As a rule, I would suggest a piece of fresh fruit as a dessert.

Some of the breakfast recipes could be used as a dessert, as could a spoonful or two of unsweetened Greek yoghurt or crème fraîche with some fresh fruit or chopped nuts. Otherwise, save desserts for occasional treats or when eating out. Try to restrict yourself to a small portion if you are going to indulge, but if not, enjoy it and accept that your glucose level will rise afterwards.

ACKNOWLEDGEMENTS

I am grateful to the many readers of *Reverse Your Diabetes – The step-by-step plan to take control of type 2 diabetes*, who took the time to contact me personally or who posted reviews online, explaining how the book had helped them. It is hugely satisfying as a doctor to know that my first effort at writing a book has helped people with diabetes make lifestyle changes that have significantly improved their ability to control their condition.

This second book moves on from the 'what' to the 'how' of making changes to one's diet, by building upon the general advice and providing a set of brand-new recipes. For these I am hugely indebted to Jonathan Hayden, who researched, tried and tested so many of the recipes. Special thanks must go to Dr Trudi Deakin, founder and chief executive of X-PERT Health, whose skills as a dietitian proved invaluable in helping ensure that the recipes in this book are balanced and appropriate. Shanta Panesar at diabetes.co.uk researched

the nutritional values of the recipes and found www.
caloriescount.com invaluable. Any mistakes, of course,
rest firmly with me. I also gratefully acknowledge the
contribution of Ute Linnenkamp of the International
Diabetes Federation, who drew together the evidence of
the links between certain foods and development of type
2 diabetes (summarised in the table on pages 33–34).

APPENDIX 1

BODY MASS INDEX GUIDANCE CHART

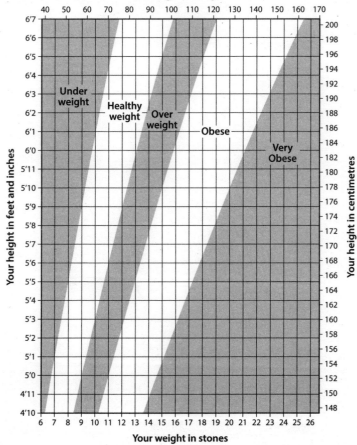

Your weight in kilograms

Under weight

Healthy weight

Over weight

Obese

Very Obese

Your height in feet and inches

Your height in centimetres

Your weight in stones

APPENDIX 2

BLOOD GLUCOSE RECORD CHARTS

Individual Meal Blood Glucose Record Chart

Date	Time	Blood glucose level before meal	Blood glucose level 2 hours after meal	After-meal blood glucose on target (y/n)?	Notes, e.g. any changes made to recipe or portion size

Daily Meal Blood Glucose Record Chart

	Meal/recipe page no	Pre-meal blood glucose	Post-meal blood glucose	Notes
Day 1	Date:			
Breakfast				
Lunch				
Dinner				
Bedtime				
Day 2	Date:			
Breakfast				
Lunch				
Dinner				
Bedtime				
Day 3	Date:			
Breakfast				
Lunch				
Dinner				
Bedtime				

APPENDIX 3

USEFUL WEBSITES

Diabetes.co.uk

Diabetes.co.uk is the UK's largest and fastest-growing community website and forum for people with diabetes:

Get support at **www.diabetes.co.uk/forum**

Like us on Facebook **www.facebook.com/Diabetes.co.uk**

Sign up for FREE Newsletter **www.diabetes.co.uk/welcome**

Buy diabetes products and accessories online **www.diabetes.co.uk/shop**

Diabetes Support Forum UK

The diabetes-support.org.uk forum is open to ALL people who want to discuss diabetes, and everyone is very welcome, but our focus is mainly on the UK NHS system.

www.diabetes-support.org.uk

International Diabetes Federation

The global advocate for people with diabetes. The mission of IDF is to promote diabetes care, prevention and a cure worldwide.

www.idf.org

Diabetes UK

The UK's leading diabetes charity. They care for, connect with and campaign on behalf of all people affected by and at risk of diabetes in local communities across the UK.
www.diabetes.org.uk

NHS Choices

Information from the National Health Service on conditions, treatments, local services and healthy living.
www.nhs.uk/Conditions/Diabetes/Pages/Diabetes.aspx

Public Library of Science

Non-profit organization of scientists committed to making the world's scientific and medical literature freely accessible to scientists and to the public.
www.plos.org

Diabetes Community

An international community for people with diabetes.
www.diabetescommunity.com

Glycaemic index

www.glycemicindex.com

Carbs and Cals

Make carb and calorie counting easy to understand and accessible to everyone.
www.carbsandcals.com

Carbohydrate counting programme

Developed by the Bournemouth Diabetes and Endocrine Centre – mainly for people on insulin.

www.bdec-e-learning.com

The NHS Diabetic Eye Screening Programme (NDESP)

The NHS Diabetic Eye Screening Programme (NDESP) aims to reduce the risk of sight loss among people with diabetes by the early detection and treatment, if needed, of sight-threatening retinopathy.

diabeticeye.screening.nhs.uk

Patient Education programmes

www.nhs.uk/Livewell/Diabetes/Pages/Diabeteseducation.aspx

APPENDIX 4

MEAL PLANNER

The aim of this book is not to prescribe a particular diet, nor is it to suggest a set number of calories or carbohydrates that you should eat each day. Rather, the aim has been to present you with recipe ideas that enable you to try out meals with different amounts of carbohydrates so that you can learn to identify the carbohydrate intake (for each meal or per day) that best enables you to keep control of your diabetes, while enabling you to continue to enjoy the foods you like to eat.

However, in order to help you along your way, we have prepared two separate weeks of meal plans that both provide between less than 100g of carbohydrates per day. Note that week B has higher calories (1100 to 1800 per day) overall than week A (900 to 1300 per day). This is to enable readers to choose a higher or lower calorie intake. Remember that while a lower calorie intake will likely be more effective at helping you lose weight, a higher calorie intake may be more sustainable for a longer period. And when it comes to pushing your diabetes into reverse, keeping up changes to your diet in the longer term is what is important.

Note I have placed the somewhat more complicated evening meal recipes at the weekends when, theoretically, you might have more time to spend in the kitchen! And don't be afraid to 'batch cook'. Soups keep very well in the fridge and the freezer as do many dishes like moussaka and La Parmigiana di Melanzane (Aubergine Parmesan). Better to have these wonderful low carb, homemade dishes to hand rather than be tempted to order a takeaway on a Friday night.

You can also see how quickly the amount of carbohydrate in any meal can quickly rise by eating an extra bread roll or second helping.

Most of all, I do hope you enjoy the recipes while at the same time improving your health.

Meal Planner

MEAL PLAN A	BREAKFAST	LUNCH	DINNER	TOTAL CARBS (Grams)	TOTAL CALORIES
Monday	Full fat natural yogurt and fruit carbs 23g/cals 190	Sardines with a Greek-style Salad *page 92* carbs 19g/cals 393	Spanish Tortilla *page 177* carbs 21g/cals 320	63g	903
Tuesday	Scrambled Eggs *page 69* carbs 1g/cals 208	Watercress and Potato Soup *page 118* carbs 16g/cals 154 Served with A granary roll (60g) carbs 28g/cals 160	Tuna Steaks with Cucumber and Tomato-flavoured Mayonnaise *page 174* carbs 5g/cals 644	50g	1166
Wednesday	Blueberry Quinoa Breakfast *page 80* carbs 37g/cals 286	Omelette with Girolle Mushrooms *page 143* carbs 3g/cals 345	Sicilian-style Tuna *page 195* carbs 11g/cals 644	51g	1275
Thursday	Boiled Egg with one piece of brown bread toast (60g) carbs 20g/cals 120	Watercress and Potato Soup *page 118* carbs 16g/cals 154	La Parmigiana di Melanzane (Aubergine Parmesan) *page 199* carbs 18g/cals 482 Served with A ciabatta roll carbs 43g/cals 230	97g	986

Continued

MEAL PLAN A	BREAKFAST	LUNCH	DINNER	TOTAL CARBS (Grams)	TOTAL CALORIES
Friday	Full fat natural yogurt and fruit carbs 23g/cals 190	Whole Sardines with a Warm Olive and Beetroot Salad *page 95* carbs 6g/cals 627	Stir-fried Chinese Leaves *page 172* carbs 8g/cals 178	37g	995
Saturday	Smoked Salmon with Chive Scrambled Egg *page 71* carbs 1g/cals 293	Mushroom Soup *page 140* carbs 24g/cals 359	Three Bean Salad *page 167* carbs 15g/cals 380 Served with One slice of whole grain rye bread (60g) carbs 30g/cals 150	70g	1182
Sunday	Fergus Henderson's Kippers *page 88* carbs 0g/cals 357	Mushroom Soup *page 140* 24g carbs/cals 359	Moussaka *page 158* carbs 24g/cals 546	48g	1262

Meal Planner

MEAL PLAN B	BREAKFAST	LUNCH	DINNER	TOTAL CARBS (Grams)	TOTAL CALORIES
Monday	Giancarlo Caldesi's Fried Eggs with Tomato Sauce *page 73* carbs 10g/cals 396	Curried Parsnip Soup *page 120* carbs 19g/cals 275	Caponata *page 155* carbs 15g/cals 372 Served with A granary roll (60g) carbs 28g/cals 160	72g	1203
Tuesday	Poached Eggs with Vegetables *page 76* 26g/cals 280	Curried Parsnip Soup (from the fridge) carbs 19g/cals 275 Served with A granary roll (60g) carbs 28g/cals 160	Mackerel with Coriander and Chilli, Served with a Red Onion and Tomato Salad *page 205* carbs 25g/cals 1008	98g	1723
Wednesday	Full fat yogurt and fruit carbs 23g/cals 190	Spanish Tortilla *page 177* carbs 21g/cals 320	Broccoli and Chicken Gratin *page 164* carbs 33g /cals 875	77g	1385
Thursday	Scrambled Eggs *page 69* carbs 1g/cals 208 And One piece of brown bread toast (60g) carbs 20g/cals 120	La Parmigiana di Melanzane (Aubergine Parmesan) *page 199* (from the freezer) carbs 18g/cals 482 Served with One piece of brown bread (60g) carbs 20g/cals 120	Caesar Salad *page 138* carbs 5g /cals 234	65g	1164

Continued

MEAL PLAN B	BREAKFAST	LUNCH	DINNER	TOTAL CARBS (Grams)	TOTAL CALORIES
Friday	Full fat yogurt and fruit carbs 23g/cals 190	Tomato Soup *page 114* carbs 23g/cals 185 Served with A granary roll (60g) carbs 28g/cals 160	Halibut *en papillote page 216* carbs 2g/cals 440 Served with Buttered Spinach carbs 4g/cals 130	80g	1105
Saturday	Omelette with Girolle Mushrooms *page 143* carbs 2.4g/cals 345	Tomato Soup (from the fridge) carbs 23g/cals 185	Kozhi Kurumulagu (Spicy Southern Indian Black Pepper Chicken) *page 186* carbs 18g/ cals 586 Served with One Mini Naan Bread carbs 29g/ cals 172	73g	1288
Sunday	Wheat-free Pancakes with Greek Yoghurt and Fruit *page 84* carbs 7g/cals 614	Smoked Mackerel Salad *page 153* carbs 18g/cals 770	Calf's Liver with Sage *page 197* carbs 13g/cals 377 Served with Broccoli and Cauliflower carbs 15g/cals 75	53g	1836

NOTES

Chapter 1: What is type 2 diabetes?

1. The UK Prospective Diabetes Study (UKPDS) was a landmark randomised, multicentre trial of glycaemic therapies in 5,102 people with newly diagnosed type 2 diabetes. It ran for 20 years (1977 to 1997) in 23 UK clinical sites and showed conclusively that the complications of type 2 diabetes, previously often regarded as inevitable, could be reduced by improving blood glucose and/or blood pressure control. The UKPDS was designed and run by the late Professor Robert Turner and Professor Rury Holman. http://www.dtu.ox.ac.uk/ukpds_trial/

2. http://www.diabetes.org/diabetes-basics/statistics/

3. http://www.niddk.nih.gov/health-information/health-statistics/Pages/overweight-obesity-statistics.aspx

4. Matthews, DR, Matthews, PC, 'Type 2 diabetes as an infectious disease: is this the black death of the 21st century?', *Diabetes Medicine* 28, (2011), 2–9

5. Taylor, R, 'Type 2 diabetes etiology and reversibility', *Diabetes Care*, 36, (2013), 1047

6. Diabetes Prevention Program Research Group, 'Reduction in the incidence of type 2 diabetes with lifestyle intervention

or metformin', *New England Journal of Medicine*, 346, (2002) 393–403

7. Lindstrom, J, Erikkson, J, Louheranta, A et al., 'The Finnish diabetes prevention study (DPS)', *Diabetes Care*, 26 (2003), 3230–3236

8. Franco, M, Bilal, U, Ordumez, P et al., 'Population-wide weight loss and regain in relation to diabetes burden and cardiovascular mortality in Cuba 1980–2010: repeated cross sectional surveys and ecological comparison of secular trends', *BMJ*, 346, (2013), f1515, doi: 10.1136/bmj.f1515

9. Guidone, C, Manco, M et al., 'Mechanisms of recovery from type 2 diabetes after malabsorptive bariatric surgery', *Diabetes*, 55, (2006)

10. Lim, EL, Hollingsworth, KG, Taylor, E et al., 'Reversal of type 2 diabetes: normalisation of beta cell function in association with decreased pancreas and liver triacylglycerol', *Diabetologia*, 54, (2011), 2506–2514

Chapter 2

1. http://openheart.bmj.com/content/2/1/e000196.full.pdf+html?sid=0ce688cf-9caa-4778-9119-996d1fd17c0e

Chapter 3

1. Ley, S, Handy, O, Wu, F; 'Prevention and management of type 2 diabetes: dietary components and nutritional strategies,' *Lancet*, 2014, 383: 1999–2007

2. Halton TL, Willett WC, Liu S, Manson JE, Stampfer MJ, Hu FB, 'Potato and french fry consumption and risk of type 2 diabetes in women.' *American Journal of Clinical Nutrition*, (Feb. 2006) 83(2): 284–90

3. Estruch, R, Ros, E, Salas-Salvado, J et al., 'Primary prevention of cardiovascular disease with a Mediterranean diet', *New England Journal of Medicine*, 368, (2013), 1279–1290

INDEX

Index

List of recipes by grams of carbohydrates

Simple breakfasts and brunches	Page no.	Carb (g)
Fergus Henderson's kippers	88	0
Scrambled eggs	69	1
Smoked salmon with chive scrambled eggs	71	1
Baked eggs with mushrooms	78	3
Wheat-free pancakes with greek yoghurt and fruit	84	7
Giancarlo Caldesi's fried eggs with tomato sauce	73	10
Pepper, ham and tomato omelette	86	10
Poached eggs with vegetables	76	26
Baked figs with goat's cheese and balsamic vinegar glaze	82	27
Blueberry quinoa breakfast	80	37
Light Lunches, Salads and Soups		
Crab on avocado with coriander-infused olive oil and herb salad	89	9
Grilled mackerel with white wine vinegar	202	0
Omelette with girolle mushrooms	143	3
Caesar salad	138	5
Sunflower seed crackers	101	5
Whole sardines with a warm olive and beetroot salad	95	6
Kidneys with white cabbage, garlic, parsley and butter	103	8
Cauliflower with onion and tomato	126	8
Chicken and vegetable soup	135	14
Broken sardines with an avocado and fennel salad	97	15
Watercress and potato soup	118	16
Vegetable curry – as you like it	129	16
Traditional tarka dal	123	16
Smoked mackerel salad	153	18
Salami with celeriac hash browns	131	19
Sardines with a greek-style salad	92	19
Curried parsnip soup	120	19
(Sort of) german lentil soup	111	19
Tomato salad	180	19
An Italian tuna salad	148	20
Lamb and leek broth	108	20
Black and kidney bean soup	133	21
Avocado and bean salad	150	22

Light Lunches, Salads and Soups	Page no.	Carb (g)
Tomato soup	114	23
Mushroom soup	140	24
Toasted goat's cheese with an avocado, pear and walnut salad	105	24
Avocado baked with egg and chorizo	99	26
Salade niçoise	145	40
Main Meals		
Halibut *en papillote*	216	2
The perfect roast cod	209	4
Tuna steaks with cucumber and tomato-flavoured mayonnaise	174	5
Poached salmon	211	5
Monkfish with saffron sauce	193	6
Pan-fried mackerel served with cucumber and chilli tagliatelle	207	6
Stir-fried chinese leaves	172	. 8
Sicilian-style tuna	195	11
Calf's liver with sage	197	13
Pan-fried Dover sole	214	13
Caponata	155	15
Three bean salad	167	15
Kozhi kurumulagu (spicy southern Indian black pepper chicken)	186	18
La parmigiana di melanzane (aubergine parmesan)	199	18
Ratatouille	162	19
Spanish tortilla	177	21
Navarin of lamb (navarin printanier)	183	22
Moussaka	158	24
Mackerel with coriander and chilli, served with a red onion and tomato salad	205	25
Chilli con carne	169	26
Broccoli and chicken gratin	164	33
Couscous made my neighbour's way	190	40